"Sara Rosenquist's take on postpartum depression is revelatory and full of hope. Her message is that what we believe shapes our biology as much as the other way around. With this new understanding, we can get back in the driver's seat. We can choose our behavior, make plans, and acquire healthy habits of body and mind. In doing so, we can shape our own mental health destiny."

—Ethan Watters, author of *Crazy Like Us*

"There are few ambitious, successful, and comprehensive guides to postpartum depression for non-experts. Fortunately for us, Rosenquist opens a path for ordinary couples to self-heal. Using direct, lucid prose and everyday examples, the author identifies and provides ways to relieve the distress of postpartum depression. I admire this book for its brilliant melding of compassionate insight, fascinating research summarizations, and presentation of exercises, chapter-by-chapter, to restore a sense of well-being."

—Elaine Crovitz, Ph.D., emeritus faculty at
Duke University Medical School

"*After the Stork* is a detailed and thoughtful guide to the challenges that new parents encounter as they make this major life transition. It offers a wealth of different practical strategies that can be used by parents to minimize or mitigate postpartum depression. Because it is so evenhanded and thorough in addressing issues that both mothers and fathers may face, it is a must-read for couples expecting or welcoming their first child."

—James F. Paulson, Ph.D., child and family clinical
psychologist and associate professor at Eastern Virginia
Medical School

"I am a female OB/GYN physician and a mother of four. After reading this book, I have insight that may help me not only be a better mom and wife, but also a better doctor. I appreciate Sara Rosenquist teaching us why depression can set in after having a child, but I also value her detailed steps and advice on how to prevent and overcome it. I will recommend this book to all my patients and friends."

> —Andrea Lukes, MD, OB/GYN physician at the Women's Wellness Clinic in Durham, NC

"Books for professionals are often long on science and short on practicality, while those for non-professionals are often filled with advice not based on scientific facts. In *After the Stork*, Rosenquist has blended the best of both worlds. Professionals will learn about the daily realities of postpartum depression, and readers with new babies will not only get exceptionally sensible guidance, but will discover the science behind it in a format that is fascinating and easy to grasp. This is a must-read for those who care for new parents, and can serve as an invaluable roadmap for those who wish to prevent or overcome postpartum depression."

> —John C. Linton, Ph.D., ABPP, professor and vice chair of the department of behavioral medicine and psychiatry at the West Virginia University School of Medicine in Charleston, VA

"The information in *After the Stork* is empowering and practical, and offers couples and prospective parents a 360-degree view of the ways in which their lives will change, both positively and negatively, after the birth or adoption of their child. Not only does she offer them knowledge, which is potent in and of itself, but she provides clear and readily accessible exercises and strategies for proactively and reactively managing issues and problems that can—and will—arise in the postpartum period."

> —Catherine A. Forneris, Ph.D., ABPP, licensed psychologist and associate professor of psychiatry at University of North Carolina at Chapel Hill

"Rosenquist has written an incredibly helpful and comprehensive handbook for couples entering into the new world of parenthood. She thoughtfully and honestly describes many of the challenges that couples encounter during pregnancy and postpartum, including postpartum depression. This workbook is an invaluable guide for couples willing to invest some time and energy into preparing for parenthood and the inevitable lifestyle adjustments that come along with it."

—Samantha Meltzer-Brody, MD, MPH,
director of the University of North Carolina
Perinatal Psychiatry Program

"In an age when pills are all too often relied upon as the first solution to life's difficulties, Rosenquist offers a refreshing, evidence-based, psychological approach to the serious problem of postpartum depression."

—Irving Kirsch, author of *The Emperor's New Drugs*

"Rosenquist has written an eminently practical book about depression, especially appropriate for men and women embarking on parenthood. She provides interesting scientific data about depression, case studies of parents struggling with postpartum depression, and explains the concrete, practical things readers can do to both prevent depression and to help treat it. Seldom do you see a mental health book that is so realistic, understandable, and scientifically interesting. From years of clinical practice, she shares simple approaches to help parents and anyone who struggles with depression."

—John F. Wilson. Ph.D., professor at the University
of Kentucky College of Medicine

after the stork

the couple's guide to preventing and overcoming postpartum depression

SARA ROSENQUIST, PH.D.

New Harbinger Publications, Inc.

Publisher's Note

This publication is designed to provide accurate and authoritative information in regard to the subject matter covered. It is sold with the understanding that the publisher is not engaged in rendering psychological, financial, legal, or other professional services. If expert assistance or counseling is needed, the services of a competent professional should be sought.

Distributed in Canada by Raincoast Books

Copyright © 2010 by Sara E. Rosenquist
New Harbinger Publications, Inc.
5674 Shattuck Avenue
Oakland, CA 94609
www.newharbinger.com

FSC
Mixed Sources
Product group from well-managed
forests and other controlled sources
Cert no. SW-COC-002283
www.fsc.org
© 1996 Forest Stewardship Council

RAINFOREST ALLIANCE
CERTIFIED

Acquired by Jess O'Brien; Cover design by Amy Shoup; Edited by Carole Honeychurch

Library of Congress Cataloging-in-Publication Data
Rosenquist, Sara E.
  After the stork : the couple's guide to preventing and overcoming postpartum depression / Sara E. Rosenquist ; foreword by Michael D. Yapko.
    p. cm.
  Includes bibliographical references.
  ISBN 978-1-57224-863-2
  1. Postpartum depression--Popular works. I. Title.
  RG852.R675 2010
  618.7'6--dc22
                              2010025664

12 11 10   10 9 8 7 6 5 4 3 2 1   First printing

This book is dedicated to my own two highly imperfect parents, from one highly imperfect daughter, and to Mary and Emily who have taught me everything I know about being a mother.

Para todos los hijos de mi alma: Emily, and Andrew and Julia, and Julie, and Guillaume, and Gimena, and Hanako, and Gaia. For all those of the younger generation who occupy space in my heart: may the challenges of parenthood yet to come bring you infinite blessings.

Contents

Foreword

When you see a happy mother and father playing with their baby, talking to him or her in that sing-song voice accompanied by obvious expressions of pleasure on their faces, you are witnessing one of the most magical moments possible in human relationships. Remarkable things are happening within the brains and bodies of each family member, and vitally important things are happening in the relationships between them that will have a profound impact on their individual lives as well as their lives together as a family.

In stark contrast, what happens when depressed moms and dads just can't find it in themselves to offer a smiling face, do the sing-song bit, hold, or even just make eye contact with the baby? The negative consequences are shared by mothers, fathers, and babies, but the impact on the newborn is especially serious. Normal brain development requires an involved parent regularly stimulating that brain through play and a rich array of interactions. Likewise, normal social, physical, and behavioral development requires parents to fully and meaningfully engage with their child. A mother lost in the abyss of postpartum depression suffers, but so does the baby she is too detached from to effectively parent. A father too preoccupied with how bad he feels to engage with his baby can go on despairing, but his baby may pay an even greater price for his suffering than he does.

The time leading up to and immediately following the birth of a child is an extraordinarily sensitive time in the lives of babies and their parents. The relationship between the mother and father undergoes a huge transition, and the quality of the relationship with the newborn will have enduring effects that can quite literally last a lifetime. That is why it is so critically important to do all you can to prevent post-partum depression when possible or respond to it as quickly and effectively as you can if it develops. Dr. Sara Rosenquist, an expert on postpartum depression, has used her extensive experience to write this frank and practical book to help readers reduce the likelihood of post-partum depression and to minimize its negative effects if and when it surfaces.

To her credit, Dr. Rosenquist has taken a much broader view of postpartum depression than experts have done previoulsy. She pro-vides compelling reasons to think of postpartum depression as some-thing much more than just biochemistry run amok; she considers psychological as well as social factors that contribute to the onset of postpartum depression. She makes the point clearly that a multidi-mensional problem can't be effectively treated in a one-dimensional way. She considers insightfully the roles of unrealistic expectations, distorted thinking, and even sexual and financial pressures on the quality of one's relationship with one's co-parent as well as with the baby. The range of topics she offers helpful advice on is impressive. Dr. Rosenquist is supportive and encouraging in her approach to this delicate subject, and she regularly reminds readers there's a great deal they can do to rise above the pit of postpartum despair.

Dr. Rosenquist helps break new ground when she speaks to the issue of the prevention of postpartum depression. She encourages readers to *think ahead*, the essential foundation of prevention. Thinking ahead, however, often sounds easier than it really is: people are typically so focused on getting through the next five minutes that it's difficult for them to think further ahead than that. Not every challenge can be anticipated and managed preventively, of course. But Dr. Rosenquist draws our attention to the issues that commonly derail individuals and couples, then provides sensible and practical advice for managing them effectively as a vital tool of prevention. Her optimistic belief that we can all do more to prevent postpartum depression is motivating. This is one of the many strengths evident in this book.

Dr. Rosenquist offers plenty of things to think about, but she also provides readers with things to *do*. The exercises she includes will help you clarify your ideas, think through ways to better handle whatever challenges you might be facing, and develop many of the key skills you'll need to live and parent well. This is not only motivating, it's empowering.

I have spent my professional life studying the disorder of depression and writing about the things people can do to acquire those skills known to reduce and even prevent depression. Thus, I have a special appreciation for the clarity and wisdom of Dr. Rosenquist's ideas and suggestions about dealing with postpartum depression. There is no overstating how important it is to have parents who are up to the tough job of parenting. Parenting isn't ever easy, by any means, but Dr. Rosenquist has certainly contributed much to make it easier—and more effective.

    —Michael D. Yapko, Ph.D.
     www.yapko.com

Introduction

Depression is a nasty experience. It is like a thick film of dark, sticky flypaper that settles over the soul, robbing a person of joy and enthusiasm. Depression colors everything, leaving little room for light and hope to enter. And because it is so very dark and so very sticky, it can also be lethal. Even when a depressed person is not suicidal, even when he or she manages to drag through life, the experience is draining and the struggle touches many others. People who are depressed infect the people around them with their joylessness. Babies look to Mom and Dad for evidence that they are loved and lovable and for cues about how to be with other human beings. And when Mom or Dad is depressed, these babies get precious little information that leads them to believe that they can make people smile. Depression is a huge drain on individuals, on families, on communities, and on society. But depression doesn't have to be—it *can* be prevented.

A New Perspective on Depression

I wrote this book because depression is a growing problem in our society, a problem that we have created and are quickly exporting all over the globe, a problem that we, as a society, have a shared responsibility for fixing. Other books on the subject emphasize the biological aspects of depression as a way of legitimating a very real problem and letting people off the hook of self-blame (a hook that really does no one any good). In *After the Stork,* I will present a different framework for understanding and explaining negative emotional experiences. Part of this new way of looking at what leads to and sustains depression is considering the context of mental illness. In other words, seeing depression as a biological, pathological mental disease can actually serve to perpetuate it, leaving real solutions untried. I undertook this project because I believe that a more accurate, nuanced understanding of depression can help us take responsibility without trafficking in blame, and by taking responsibility, by looking in all of the *right* places, begin to find solutions that offer lasting hope and lasting help. I also believe that if we can catch depression when it first happens—which often is after the first really big transition in life, the transition to parenthood—we can prevent a lot of misery and perhaps even protect our children from developing a vulnerability to depression in the future.

If you are willing to take an honest look at yourself, this book can be of great value. In it I'll offer the tools to identify and change habits of thinking that you're probably not aware of, habits that are so automatic and so ingrained that you wouldn't otherwise have any reason to question them. If you're willing to make yourself vulnerable to self-awareness without resorting to self-recrimination, this book can also offer you many tips for improving your relationships and for making choices that balance what's good for you with what's good for others. Instead of looking to biology as the starting point or root cause of depression, I invite you to consider that habits of thought and habits of relating are equally valid starting points. Changes in either of these groups of habits can result in very real, measurable changes to your brain and biochemistry. With this new, interlocking, circular view of cause and effect, we can begin to make small changes on multiple fronts simultaneously. These are the changes that offer real hope for ending the misery and beginning to construct a vibrant life of optimism, mutual support, and connection to community.

The Origins of This Book

This book began twenty-six years ago as my dissertation. I was newly married at the time and considering when to start my own family. The topic of postpartum depression was relatively new then, and the operative questions about it revolved around how stress and social support work together to create vulnerabilities to depression or to protect people from depression. I noticed the total omission of fathers from this research and zeroed in on it. But I wasn't prepared for the results: roughly equal numbers of moms and dads get depressed after the birth of a baby. The graphs of the data demonstrated a perfect function of high stress plus low spousal support for each parent.

Between writing the proposal and defending my dissertation, I got pregnant and had my baby—along with my own initiation into the dark, hollow experience of this thing we classify as a mood disorder. And since that time, I've raised my daughter, changed my habits of thought, become more intentional about my habits of relating, and accumulated hundreds of hours of advanced training and thousands of hours of clinical experience. I've submitted samples of my work to the scrutiny of my most distinguished colleagues, and I've received the highest credentials of my profession. Both as a professional and as a mother, I know whereof I speak. I know the sleepless nights and despairing moments and the useless self-recrimination and endless loops of frustration. My hope is to relieve you of these burdens by providing a clear map of the territory and practical strategies for its safe travel.

The Path, in Brief

After the Stork begins with an examination of what scientists call the *bio-psycho-social model* of mental health and illness. After decades of research about which is most important, nature or nurture, we in the scientific community have been forced to conclude that all of human experience is the result of a complex interplay of biological, psychological, and social (including cultural) factors. But old notions of the duality of conscious and unconscious mind, of mind and body, and old linear notions of cause and effect continue to get in the way of accurate understanding and helpful explanations. So please read these beginning chapters slowly and carefully. I ask that you approach this information with an attitude of curiosity about how your own most deeply held assumptions might catch you by surprise or shape your responses. I suspect that reading with a notebook and pencil close at hand will help you get the greatest benefit. If you're like me, you might be tempted to just read through the book with the idea of going back a second time to jot down questions and comments or to make notes about what might be helpful. As I've discovered, we often find ourselves swept away in the undertow of life, never to return to the closer reading we promised ourselves we'd accomplish. That's why, in order to get the most benefit from this book, you'll probably do well to start out with the notebook and pencil nearby from the get-go.

After carefully explaining the research that supports our understanding of the bio-psycho-social model of depression, I go on to discuss the ways in which our modern culture has created a vortex of vulnerability for new parents: as parents in our culture, we are encouraged to believe and hold expectations about parenthood that simply cannot coexist with the intensity of work demands and the contradictory pressures we've created for ourselves. Then we'll examine how sleep and sex are affected by new parenthood and discuss what you can do to protect these two areas of your life—areas that can serve a vital, restorative function that helps protect against depression. The final two chapters will help you gain perspective and learn strategies for managing two of the most common sources of stress in our society—parenting and finances.

Depression varies a great deal, and the areas of life that people experience as most stressful—most straining of mental, emotional, interpersonal, and financial resources—vary widely. Thus some chapters will be more helpful for some readers than for others. I hope you will take care to read the first three chapters in order, and then feel free to sample from the advice chapters as best fits your situation, guided by your unique set of interests and needs.

A New Season of Life

Our children are only babies once. However stressful this time might be, it's important to remember that it will pass quickly. Try to remember that today's bewilderment will one day be the stuff of all your funny baby stories. For instance, I still think about the time I drove to the grocery store with my four-month-old daughter strapped into her car seat. In a great burst of brilliance (motivated by the desire to be efficient), I decided to get the car locked up. That way, I wouldn't have to fumble with my keys while holding my tiny baby (this was before people had automatic locking devices). Dropping my keys onto the passenger seat, I pushed down the lock button next to the passenger side, then on the driver's side. Getting out and turning to get the baby out of her carseat, I slammed my door. As I heard the door engage, I saw my car keys still on the passenger seat. Uh oh. I realized in horror that I had locked my baby girl in and myself out. Very efficient—not very helpful.

Parenting is a wonderful season of life, but it will be much more enjoyable if you approach it with self-forgiveness, an acceptance of your feelings, and humor. And the lessons you learn in this season can help you learn good habits that will serve you and your family well your whole life long. The habits of thought and the habits of relating that you learn and practice now will be the practices that you model for your children, habits that will protect them from depression and help them go on to create a vibrant, joyful life of their own.

So, if you are ready to take a look at yourself, if you're prepared to make some difficult choices, let's get started. Go ahead and roll up your sleeves, settle into a comfortable chair, and begin to read, notebook and pencil at hand. Sift carefully. Consider what applies to you, try out some new strategies, reach out to other parents, and stay connected to your partner. May this book and the ideas it contains help you really enjoy your new baby.

CHAPTER 1

Postpartum Depression: More Than Just Hormones

A lie can travel halfway around the world while the truth is putting on its shoes.

Mark Twain

Most likely, you've picked up this book because you or your partner recently gave birth. You're tired, you may be worried, and you're feeling depressed. Well, if you're a woman who has recently become a mother and you're feeling very down, it must be postpartum depression, right? Those hormones can really do a number on you—that's what everyone says. So you're just going to have to wait until the hormones even out and then you (or your partner) will be back to normal again.

But let's take a moment to imagine that the new baby hasn't come into *your* life. Let's imagine that the couple living in the apartment next to yours just had the baby. The infant is up most of the nights crying, and the wall separating your bedroom and theirs is flimsy. It seems as though the baby is right in your bedroom. Whereas before you used to get a solid seven hours of sleep a night, now you're getting at most three or four, in choppy fits.

On top of this (and no doubt exacerbated by it), you and your spouse have been fighting more than usual. In addition, lately you've had much less time for yourself than you used to—you just got a new puppy, who is turning out to be more demanding than you had expected. You're spending at least an hour in the morning before work and an hour or two in the evenings taking care of her and calming her down—time that you used to enjoy jogging, reading, and chatting with your spouse (in the days before you two were fighting so much.)

Just when you thought things couldn't get any worse, some major unexpected repairs need to be done on your home at your expense, effectively cutting into your disposable income by 30 percent or more overnight. You have less money for movies, eating out, and new clothes, and sometimes you even wonder how you are going to pay routine expenses like your phone and electricity bills.

Finally, a major goal you had, something you had been looking forward to your whole life—perhaps finishing writing a novel or reaching an executive-level position in your job—has just come to fruition, and you're finding that all the fulfillment you had hoped it would bring isn't there. Life is pretty much the same as it always was except that rest, leisure, and fun are now harder to come by.

If you found yourself in these unfortunate circumstances, could you imagine that all of these stresses taken together might possibly bring you down? Do you suppose that this combination of events might even trigger clinical depression? Millions of American women and men find themselves in circumstances very much like these every year. They're called new mothers and fathers. The transition to parenthood is not simple anymore; our lives are too full and too complicated. But you don't have to wait for your "hormones to settle down," and you don't have to do this alone. You can read this book, take notes, and talk to your partner; you can be compassionate both with yourself and with your family about your situation *and* that you can act to heal yourself.

Defining Depression

So what is depression, anyway? The American Psychiatric Association publishes the definitive catalogue of mental disorders, called the

Diagnostic and Statistical Manual of Mental Disorders or DSM. The manual is constantly under study and in the process of being revised to conform to the latest research findings. It is currently in its fourth revised version. Before 1980, the DSM had included a separate category for postpartum depression. But in the 1980 revision (the DSM III), this entry was removed. Recent research had found that, once a person is depressed, the symptoms, biochemistry, and treatment are the same no matter what particular vulnerability or combination of vulnerabilities might have triggered the depression (Purdy and Frank 1993). In other words, depression is depression, postpartum or not.

According to the DSM-IVTR, *depression* is first of all a mood disorder—a major mental illness (2000). The symptoms of depression include:

- Sadness, anxiety, or "empty" feelings

- Decreased energy, fatigue, being "slowed down"

- Loss of interest or pleasure in activities that were once enjoyed, including sex

- Insomnia, oversleeping, or waking much earlier than usual

- Loss of weight or appetite, or overeating and weight gain

- Feelings of hopelessness and pessimism

- Feelings of helplessness, guilt, and worthlessness

- Thoughts of death or suicide, or suicide attempts

- Difficulty concentrating, making decisions, or remembering

- Restlessness, irritability, or excessive crying

- Chronic aches and pains or physical problems that do not respond to treatment

The National Institute of Mental Health (NIMH) reported in 1999 that about 20 million Americans suffer from depression. In the general population, about 3 percent to 5 percent of men and 7 percent to 10 percent of women are depressed at any given time (Paulson, Dauber, and Leiferman 2006).

A Word About Professional Help

Depression is always a potentially serious condition; it is the leading cause of suicide, after all. So it's important that depression not be ignored or taken lightly. When the vegetative symptoms of sleep and appetite disturbance and the inability to experience pleasure accompany persistent low mood, when a person starts thinking that death could be a reasonable escape and despair takes root, then it's time to put down self-help guides and get professional help. My greatest hope is that people reading this book will be able to identify the patterns that predispose them to depression and thereby prevent it. But if you're already depressed, this is no time to try your hand at do-it-yourself fixes. Depression is very treatable, and once you know the secret combination, you can use what you learn in therapy to keep it from happening again. But the key is to get competent professional help sooner rather than later. Every moment you spend depressed is a moment lost—and it doesn't have to be that way.

A Broader View: Getting the Whole Picture on Postpartum Depression

While the stress of events such as those I've described could easily explain a great deal of the depression that commonly occurs postpartum, medical professionals and pop culture as a whole generally attribute postpartum depression strictly to hormones, regardless of social and environmental factors.

For example, in 2009, the leading nonprofit organization promoting mental health awareness, Mental Health America, posted the following on their educational website: *"Mothers commonly experience what is called 'the baby blues,' mood swings that are the result of high hormonal fluctuations that occur during and immediately after childbirth"* (nmha.org/go/information/get-info/depression/postpartum-disorders*).*

And this is what the government site on women's health pulls up regarding postpartum depression (womenshealth.gov/faq/depression-pregnancy.cfm):

> After pregnancy, hormonal changes in a woman's body may trigger symptoms of depression. During pregnancy, the amount of two female hormones, estrogen and progesterone, in a woman's body increases greatly. In the first twenty-four hours after childbirth, the amount of these hormones rapidly drops back down to their normal nonpregnant levels. Researchers think the fast change in hormone levels may lead to depression, just as smaller changes in hormones can affect a woman's moods before she gets her menstrual period (2009).

In short, they tell us that hormonal fluctuation is the reason women get depressed after childbirth. But, when you think about it, there are some problems with this cut-and-dried view. Women have been having babies since the beginning of time, and we can safely assume that the hormonal changes that accompany pregnancy and childbirth have remained constant. These fluctuations are a normal part of the process of becoming a mother. Why should we believe that these normal hormonal changes would also be the single cause of depression, a full-fledged mental disorder that only afflicts *some* parents? Moreover, to imagine that biochemistry *alone* can account for something as complex as how a couple adjusts to parenthood is necessarily limiting and may prevent us from seeing the full scope of the problem—and its solutions.

The Power of Culture

Our Western medical establishment has long assumed that mental illness is mostly unaffected by culture, that expressions of brain pathology and chemical imbalances are identical the world over. Ethan Watters recently addressed this assumption in his book *Crazy Like Us: The Globalization of the American Psyche* (2010) and in an essay in the *New York Times*, "The Americanization of Mental Illness" (January 8, 2010), adapted from his book. Watters argues that "Western mental-health practitioners often prefer to believe that the 844 pages of the

DSM-IV ... describe real disorders of the mind, illnesses with symptomatology and outcomes relatively unaffected by shifting cultural beliefs." In other words, diseases of the mind are not at all like diabetes, or strep, or syphilis, or polio, or other medical problems because mental illness is inseparable from the beliefs we use to understand our experience and inseparable from the culture that shapes those beliefs (Watters 2010). For example, not everyone who experiences a traumatic event goes on to develop post-traumatic stress disorder; some people grow in positive ways after trauma, and new evidence is beginning to emerge that Hispanics experience different symptoms of PTSD than do Caucasians when they do develop the disorder (Meiser-Stedman et al. 2009; Marshall, Schell, and Miles 2009; Hefferon, Grealy, and Mutrie 2009).

Many people bristle at the notion that how we *think* about our experience actually *shapes* it, hearing truth as blame and reacting defensively by recoiling and lashing out. But Watters does not mean to dismiss suffering as psychosomatic or to blame the victims of disorders as malingers or fantasists. The fact that *what* we believe, *how* we think about our experience, actually *shapes* our experience "does not mean that these illnesses and the pain associated with them are not real, or that sufferers deliberately shape their symptoms to fit a certain cultural niche. It means that a mental illness is an illness of the mind and cannot be understood without understanding the ideas, habits, and predispositions—the idiosyncratic cultural trappings—of the mind that is its host" (Watters 2010).

Psychiatry has labored for decades to legitimate mental illness by extending the analogy to physical conditions. But this well-intended effort has ended up overstretching the analogy. Recasting mental phenomena as diseases of the brain, somehow separable from the personalities and life stories of individual sufferers, has backfired; instead of gaining, we've ended up losing much-needed perspective and losing much of value in the process. Depression itself is a relatively new idea. Gary Greenberg, a psychologist-turned-journalist, does an extraordinary job of documenting the history of the concept of depression in his book *Manufacturing Depression* (2010), a book I highly recommend for anyone desiring a more complete understanding of the diagnosis.

Once we posit that depression is inflected by culture, we can think through the hormones-only argument with cultural and historical comparison. That is, if the hormones related to pregnancy and birth were the cause of postpartum depression, then women in every culture and throughout history would also suffer from postpartum depression, while men and adoptive parents never would. Moreover, taking this thought process another step, if the hormones related to pregnancy and birth were the only cause of postpartum depression, then postpartum depression would be verifiably different from other kinds of depression—depression occurring in other people at other times in the life cycle. But it isn't. Perhaps surprisingly, women have *not* always suffered postpartum depression. Nor do women in all cultures evidence postpartum depression, while men in America do, as do adoptive parents (at about the same rates as do birth parents) (Senecky et al. 2009).

American girls and boys are taught from an early age that women's emotions, mother's moods, are a function of the menstrual cycle (Barrett and Bliss-Moreau 2009). Girls learn to pay attention to the hormonal fluctuations in their body and to dismiss or magnify their emotions accordingly. Boys learn to think of girls and women as emotional creatures driven by internal mysteries beyond their comprehension or influence. Girls grow into women, boys become men, and together they enter parenthood bracing for hormonally induced changes yet unprepared for the real challenges ahead. Meanwhile, our Western medical model of mental illness backfires—increasing the stigma of mental illness instead of reducing it (Watters 2010).

The hormonal frame, instead of bringing relief, blinds and binds. It blinds partners to the importance of connection to larger community, blinds parents to one another's struggles, limits other person perspective taking, and binds the search for solutions. Most alarmingly, instead of facilitating compassion and enabling new moms and dads to reach out to each other or to friends or professionals for help, it disconnects women from themselves and alienates couples from each other. Each spouse stands vigilant for signs of danger or unpredictability from the other; each is suspicious and distancing, binding rather than releasing the free flow of love and affection.

Moving Away from the Biological Frame

The first step in helping *all* parents with PPD—women and men, biological and adoptive, straight and gay—is to break the stranglehold that this pure-biology mindset has on the way we think about PPD. Here we will look at the whole picture; we will see how the modern hopes, expectations, and fantasies of parenthood clash with reality, setting the stage for disappointment precisely when (according to our cultural mores) disappointment is not allowed. How can anyone be disappointed when all their dreams have just come true? How indeed can one *not* be disappointed when life will never be the same and the new normal isn't clear yet? How can one not be disappointed when roles are shifting, sleep is scarce, and sex is nonexistent?

We will take a look at how sleep deprivation, particularly when complicated by certain habits of thought, predisposes one to depression and how the growing divide caused by sexual neglect can also tip the scales. We will also see how certain parenting choices, initially made in the haze of sleeplessness or well-intended tenderness, can actually make matters worse. Finally, we'll look at ways to corral runaway finances to minimize the strain on an already delicate couple system. There isn't much we can do about biology except take a pill, and the pills have fallen far short of promise (Kirsch 2010). But there *is* a great deal we can do about habits of thought, social structures, and lifestyle to ease the transition to parenthood. Human beings are hardwired to manufacture happiness out of difficult circumstances (Gilbert 2005). But in order to recover this ability we first have to see clearly through the maze of contradictory messages and perhaps let go of some favorite fantasies.

Shattering the Hormone Myth: Fathers' Experiences

Part of turning away from the idea that hormones alone cause PPD is to acknowledge information that counters that idea. For instance, what about dads who get depressed? Let's begin by taking a closer look at the situation of a pretty typical couple and their postpartum experience.

Alex and Sydney are a typical middle-class American couple. When baby Skylar was born, Sydney adjusted pretty well. She started exercising right away, and the weight she had gained during pregnancy came off fairly quickly. Skylar was an active baby, and Sydney loved being a mom. Six weeks of maternity leave went by in a flash, and Syd was back at work, juggling executive meetings and day care. But Alex wondered where his wife had disappeared to. He missed their long walks and the way they would talk about everything. Whenever he tried to be romantic, Syd seemed far away. The truth of the matter was she always had an ear out for the baby. She lived poised to jump at the slightest whimper.

Alex started staying at work later. When he came home he was either online or reaching for a beer. He had gained a lot of weight during her pregnancy. Their friends had joked that theirs was such an egalitarian marriage that they were expecting twins—Syndey carried one and Alex the other. Missing Syd and feeling left out, Alex also started working out more. Adam often thought that if sweat were tears, everyone would be able to see how deeply he hurt. Not that he didn't love Skylar—of course he did. But he missed Sydney so much that he thought his heart would break. Still, it wasn't until he realized that he was drinking just so he could get to sleep at night that he decided he'd better get some professional help.

Alex was clinically depressed. Even though he had not given birth, his depression occurred after the birth of their daughter and in response to the many changes to his life that Skylar's birth ushered in. Alex had postpartum depression. But like in many men, his depression showed more as an empty restlessness than an active sadness.

Alex could be the poster child for male postpartum depression. Although he hadn't experienced pregnancy, labor, or delivery, and although his depression looked different from the typically tearful new mom's, he was reeling from the adjustment. Hormones, as important as they may be, are clearly not the whole story. In fact, although in our modern Western culture women's emotions are commonly attributed to fluctuations in reproductive hormones, men experience just as many moods as do women. One of my favorite studies along these lines was a 1991 investigation into expectancy effects and PMS (Gallant et al. 1991). The researchers used men as the control group, assigning the men an arbitrary twenty-eight-day cycle and comparing the daily mood ratings of women to men. Although the men's moods didn't show a cyclical pattern, they *did* vary just as much as did the moods of women. And women's moods showed a cyclical pattern only when they expected them to; in other words, when they were in the part of the study where they were told that the study was about PMS (Gallant et al. 1991). Think about it: men had just as much variability in their moods over an arbitrary twenty-eight-day time period as did women throughout their cycle. Research shows that we make different attributions about women's emotions than we do about men's. When a woman shows emotion, both male and female research subjects attribute her emotion to her character ("she's emotional"), even when they have information about the situation. But when a man shows emotion, both men and women attribute his emotions to the context (Barrett and Bliss-Moreau 2009).

Couvade: Pregnancy Symptoms in Men

Before considering fathers and postpartum depression specifically, it is important to acknowledge that men and women experience emotions in response to life, and *all* emotions are biochemical and neurological events. Emotions are complex responses that occur both in the body and in the brain. Hormones are just one of many factors that can influence how we experience emotions, but, just as importantly, our emotions also influence our hormones along with other aspects of body and brain. The changes of pregnancy are obvious, so attributing a women's emotions during pregnancy and immediately afterward to hormone changes seems perfectly logical. What is less obvious is a dad can also experience physiological and even hormonal changes when his partner is pregnant and after she gives birth (Mason and Elwood 1995; Bartlett 2004; Storey et al. 2000).

Men and women in intimate partnership conceive new lives together and journey into the great life transition of parenthood. And this transition begins well before the baby is born. Perhaps most astonishingly, some men experience a kind of pregnancy. Anthropologists long ago observed that in some (usually pre-industrialized) cultures, men exhibited symptoms of pregnancy when their wives were pregnant and sometimes even went through a false labor and mock delivery in a highly ritualized form. Anthropologists dubbed this the *couvade* phenomenon, a name they got from the Basque French word *couvrir*, which means "to hatch" or "to cover." Before about 1960, Westerners regarded couvade as a deviant phenomenon, something experienced by "primitive" men and only severely neurotic or psychotic Western men (Klein 1991; Brennan et al. 2007; Conner and Denson 1990; Clinton 1986; Cohelo 1949). But in 1965, the *British Journal of Medicine* noted that gastrointestinal symptoms among men whose wives are pregnant are so common that "it is best not to regard the couvade syndrome as a psychiatric diagnosis" (Trethowan and Conlon 1965). Since then, more research has appeared showing that in fact, men—normal, nonpsychotic, Western men—commonly do experience somatic symptoms (real physical discomforts) that coincide with the pregnancy of their partner. These include "more frequent and serious episodes of colds, unintentional weight gain, numerous gastrointestinal discomforts, irritability, nervousness, inability to concentrate, headache, restlessness, excessive fatigue, and insomnia during various trimesters of pregnancy and the early postpartum period" (Clinton 1986). Fully 46 percent of expectant fathers gained weight during the first trimester and 47 percent gained weight during their partner's third trimester (Clinton 1986).

In another study, researchers looked through the medical records from a large health maintenance organization (HMO). They selected a random sample of 300 pregnancies and looked for evidence of what they called "couvade syndrome" (often referred to colloquially as simply "couvade") among the partners of these pregnant women, the expectant fathers. The definition of couvade that they used was simply that the man had sought medical attention while his wife was pregnant for symptoms that he had not sought medical attention for before she became pregnant and had not sought treatment for after she delivered (Lipkin and Lamb 1982). They found that fully 22 percent of the expectant fathers in their sample met this criterion for couvade syndrome. In other words, 22 percent of the men whose wives were pregnant had gone to their doctor complaining of things they hadn't noticed before she was pregnant and didn't notice after the baby was born. These men had twice the number of medical visits during their wife's pregnancy, they complained of twice as many symptoms, and they were significantly more likely to be prescribed medication. Although the results jumped out at the researchers, it was especially interesting that medical staff *never once* noticed the connection between a man's health complaints and his wife's pregnancy, and in fact, the records rarely mention the man being an expectant father at all (Lipkin and Lamb 1982). Medical professionals did not expect to see men in this role, so they didn't make the connection. Expectancies shape what we look for and expectancies shape how we interpret what we do see (Kirsch 1999).

The Biology of Togetherness

The men involved in the studies I mention above were clearly experiencing "biological" changes in reaction to their partner's pregnancy. Maybe those changes weren't brought about by fluctuations in estrogen or progesterone per se, but a man who experiences *couvade* or other health complaints at this time demonstrates how his social situation—his close relationship with a pregnant partner—can directly affect his biology. In the light of this construct, we can say that everything in life is "biological" and nothing is "just" biological. In other words, the social affects the emotional, which affects the biological, which affects the social, and on and on. No one factor is determinative, because each impacts the other. That's why the hormone-only theory of PPD simply doesn't hold up. To properly understand and treat PPD, we need to look at all of these factors *and how they interact.*

With this idea firmly in mind, we can begin to piece some things together. Carolyn Mason and Robert Elwood (1995) proposed that there might well be a biological underpinning to the male symptoms that constitute couvade syndrome. There is some evidence that "close contact with a pregnant partner can induce hormonal changes that enhance and accelerate the onset of paternal responsiveness in some men, as has been found in nonhuman animal studies" (Storey et al. 2000). These hormones seem to prepare men for fatherhood and encourage responsiveness to an infant: males who have never reproduced ignore, avoid, or aggress toward infants of the species. During their mates' first pregnancy, however, they show a shift toward paternal responsiveness toward all infants of their species. By the time their own young are born they are in a "paternal state" and ready to play a role in assisting in the survival of the young. This onset of paternal care is found in a variety of mammals ranging from rodents and carnivores to monkeys and gorillas (Mason and Elwood 1995). Anthropological data shows that men have moderate to high contact with infants in about 40 percent of cultures worldwide, and those are cultures where couple intimacy is high (Storey et al. 2000). Culture shapes behavior, and behavior shapes biology—which shapes behavior, which shapes culture... So much for simple cause-and-effect thinking!

In another fascinating study, Canadian researchers assessed hormone levels of men and their pregnant partners before and after the delivery of the couple's first child and measured various indices of responsiveness to infant cues. The men who had experienced couvade symptoms showed measurably higher levels of prolactin and experienced a more dramatic temporary drop in testosterone levels just after the birth (Storey et al. 2000). The researchers concluded that, "while still far from a functional proof of hormonal involvement in paternal behavior, these data nevertheless suggest that men exposed to *appropriate stimuli* undergo hormonal changes around the birth of their child that may facilitate the expression of paternal behavior" (Storey et al. 2000).

Another possibility for a biological mechanism underlying couvade-syndrome symptoms is the concept of *compathy*—the physical manifestation of empathy or what might be thought of as the "contagion" of physical distress. As an example, think of what happens when you see someone yawn. More often than not, you'll find yourself yawning too. Or, when we're near someone who is vomiting, we may respond by gagging sympathetically (Morse 1997). This physical empathy might well have its roots in the newly discovered phenomenon of mirror neurons (Gallese 2003; Rizzolatti and Craighero 2004; Iacoboni and Mazziotta 2007). *Mirror neurons* are neurons in the brains of monkeys and humans that fire not only when the animal (or person) engages in a given action, but also when said individual merely observes others engaging in the same action. These mirror neurons are now thought to be important to the neurophysiology of many behaviors essential to social survival, empathy, and emotional intelligence (Iacoboni and Dapretto 2006). What scientists don't know is *how*—how mirror neurons affect biochemistry and hormones and how behavior changes hormone levels and the number of mirror neurons making connections in the brain. What we do know is that culture shapes behavior and behavior shapes biology—biochemistry, neurochemistry, and even the neural architecture of the brain, the interconnection between neurons.

Under the Lamplight: Confirmation Bias

So, for a variety of reasons, a man experiences his partner's pregnancy emotionally, and sometimes those emotions translate into physical symptoms. Not incidentally, men also experience the birth with a wide range of emotions and biological changes as well. However, we usually don't hear much about these phenomena. Though there are studies out there about male reactions to pregnancy in a partner (as I've cited), the research is not as plentiful as you might expect for such an important experience. This lack may be because male reactions to pregnancy aren't what researchers (or those who fund them) see as significant, and research is all too often determined by the assumptions scientists hold when they define the parameters of their studies. Sometimes I think of this situation like the proverbial drunk who is looking for his keys under the lamplight. He directs his attention there not because he suspects he'll find his keys there, but because that's where the light is. It doesn't matter that his keys actually lie a block away, where it's dark. Just like the poor, keyless drunk, we often ask questions with our favorite answers in mind. So, it can come as no surprise that we get the answers we think we're looking for.

This phenomenon—getting the answers we expect to get because of the way we've framed our questions—has been dubbed by psychologists as *confirmation bias*. This tendency to see what we're looking for is supposed to be offset by the scientific method. In other words, the evidence should always point us in the correct direction. However, if we're only seeing what we expect to see, even hard evidence can sail right over our heads in favor of a comfortable and expected answer.

For instance, consider our understanding of the term "postpartum." If we define it in terms of the act of childbirth and the physical results of that act, then we get very different research findings than if we define the term postpartum in terms of a time period—the time immediately following the birth of a child. And, if when we define postpartum, we include the stress that changing roles and identity entails, we get yet another picture. The first definition limits research ahead of time. If we see the experience of postpartum as necessarily physical—stemming from the physical condition of pregnancy and the physical act of childbirth—then we'll naturally see the results in terms of biology and physicality. Therefore, postpartum difficulties are framed as manifestations of physical changes, hormonal imbalances and the like. These assumptions tend to define research questions in advance and predetermine the results. As we examine the postpartum experience, we must consider the confirmation bias for the view that women's emotions are caused by women's reproductive hormones and reproductive acts. That's the way it's been framed by much of medical science, so that's usually the result we see. End of story, right?

But what if we define the term postpartum as a time period rather than a physical state? With this broader view, we would naturally expand the focus of research to include both fathers and adoptive parents. Suddenly, we get interesting new results. In fact, we find that "postpartum" depression actually does occur in men and even in adoptive parents, neither of whom have the hormonal changes that a postpartum mother experiences.

Prevalence Rates: How Often Does PPD Happen in Dads?

Isolated research studies can be very useful in shedding light on a particular scientific question, but it takes an accumulation of studies all pointing to the same results to really provide solid conclusions. Research that combines the results of several different studies looking for much larger trends is called "meta-analysis." Meta-analytic studies show that significant numbers of new fathers experience depression after the birth of a baby (Ballard and Davies 1996; Goodman 2004).

Specifically, J. Goodman (2004) did a meta-analysis of all the then-available research into postpartum depression that included fathers. She found twenty articles that vaguely mentioned distress in fathers but only nine studies that looked specifically at postnatal depression in men. In these studies, the incidence of depression in new fathers is often not clear because of confirmation bias. But despite the relative scarcity of research specific to postpartum depression in dads,

Goodman and others (Leathers, Kelley, and Richman 1997; Wang and Chen 2006) have found that the incidence of depression in fathers hovers at around 10 percent—which is not far from the 14 percent incidence rate of postpartum depression in mothers (Paulson, Dauber, and Leiferman 2006; Paulson, Keefe, and Leiferman 2009).

While studies consistently show that about 10 percent of new fathers suffer from postpartum depression, it is perhaps even more important to note that many of these fathers continue to be depressed six weeks (Ballard et al. 1994; Ballard and Davies 1996), two months, and even six months later (Zelkowitz and Milet 2001), suggesting that because we are not identifying dads as having postpartum depression, we're not treating them. We already knew that postpartum depression in moms has a very negative impact on babies and young children (Diego et al. 2004; Sohr-Preston and Scaramella 2006; Beck 1998). However, research is just beginning to look for and show that postpartum depression in dads *also* has a negative effect on babies and children, particularly the baby's rate of language acquisition (Paulson, Dauber, and Leiferman 2006; Carro et al. 1993; Paulson, Keefe, and Leiferman 2009). Since researchers are just now getting around to studying depression in dads, we can be confident that we have only just begun to understand how a father's mood might affect an infant— we've only just now touched the tip of the iceberg. But if we can understand our own biases and step back from them, then we can begin to find more meaningful and more lasting solutions.

Why We Focus on Hormones

We've looked at how confirmation bias tends to point researchers in the direction of hormonal causes for postpartum difficulties. But how did we get to the confirmation bias in the first place? Where did we get the idea that women are controlled by their hormones, anyway?

When two events occur in a predictable sequence, it is very easy to infer that the first one caused the second. In Western cultures, women are taught to pay attention to their menstrual cycles and to their moods. Further, women are taught to attribute their moods to their menstrual cycles. Therefore, we pay close attention to each change and shift we experience throughout the month, tending to attribute many of them to our cycles. But, to attend to subtle nuances of an experience can actually shape that experience. We see and experience what we expect to see and experience.

For example, one of my clients, Amy, is a great lover of nature, and she has a particular interest in monarch butterflies. Amy has read books and attended lectures all about the monarch, so she knows that they migrate through our area, North Carolina, sometime in October. During the third week of October her spirits were lifted, and she attributed her joy to having spent a whole week surrounded by monarch butterflies. Everywhere she looked, in every tree and bush and outside every window, she saw monarch butterflies. The beauty of them inspired and comforted her. But *I* never noticed a single monarch butterfly all that week. Nor did any of the other people I spoke with. I tell Amy's story often—we notice the things we expect to notice and pay attention to what we expect to see. Amy saw the monarch butterflies the week that they migrated through North Carolina, and none of my other clients did. Life is like that.

This point was brought home for me recently when another of my clients, a young woman in her mid-twenties, reported that she had experienced all the symptoms of PMS but hadn't gotten her period. She had gone off the pill three weeks prior and expected that her body would jump right back into ovulating in the twenty-eight-day schedule she was accustomed to. She unconsciously tracked where she was in her cycle and expected PMS. She was supposed to be a week away from her period, so she felt moody and irritable. But her period never came, and no, she wasn't pregnant. Life presented the usual array of frustrations, disappointments, and challenges; but since she expected to be at a certain point in her cycle, she allowed herself to focus more on her internal states and her moods, and she attributed those naturally occurring fluctuations to her supposed cycle. Except that she really had no idea where her body was hormonally because she just came off the pill. It can take time for some women's bodies to get back into the groove of ovulating and menstruating after having been chemically paused for a period of time.

Women who give birth experience two physiological changes about three days after delivery. One is that their milk comes in, engorging the breasts and ending the flow of colostrum. The other is that levels of two hormones, estrogen and progesterone, drop suddenly and dramatically from what they were during pregnancy. This drop has been singled out as the main cause for postpartum depression. In an effort to confirm this notion, some researchers have succeeded in artificially inducing depression in women by replicating this hormonal fluctuation. They pumped the subjects up with the hormones that are typical of pregnancy, then suddenly withdrew the increased flow (Bloch et al. 2000). The result: some women got depressed. But the really interesting thing was that the only women who got depressed were ones who had been depressed before—those who had a history of depression (Bloch et al. 2000; Bloch, Daly, and Rubinow 2003).

To me, the fact that only women who had previously been depressed experienced depression when their hormones were manipulated this way strongly suggests an expectancy effect. Something about having had a history of depression made a difference, but why? I think it may be because women who have experienced depression are more likely to be internally focused, and that very internal focus is, of course, going to magnify subtle physiological changes that accompany fluctuations in reproductive hormones. An internal focus is often one of the cognitive style characteristics of depression (Yapko 1997). The tendency to attribute negative events to stable, unchangeable factors like biology is also characteristic of depression (Starr and Davila 2008; Haeffel et al. 2008; Abramson, Seligman, and Teasdale 1978). And finally, correlating hormonally associated internal states with emotions is common in our culture but not others.

In Western cultures some women experience emotional vulnerability and tearfulness when the hormones of pregnancy drop, and this state is commonly called the *new-baby blues*. But it's important to note that, according to anthropologists, this low mood is not seen in all cultures (Harkness 1987; Stern and Kruckman 1983). Anthropologists have been unable to find any evidence of the blues or any other depressive symptoms among the Kokwet people of Kenya (Harkness 1987) and have found very little evidence of postpartum depressive symptoms among Malaysian women (Kit, Janet, and Jegasothy 1997). Even among Hispanics in this country, postpartum depression rates are extraordinarily low (Wei et al. 2008). Fiji is another culture where postpartum blues, as we know it, is unheard of and postpartum depression is nonexistent. However, among Fijians there is a syndrome called *na tadoka nivasucu*, which translates as "the flu of childbirth." *Na tadoka nivasucu* is very rare and doesn't show up as tearfulness or emotional vulnerability but rather as nonspecific bodily complaints such as headache, stomachache, or toothache. It is, nonetheless, of great concern to Fijians when it does occur. Fijians know that *na tadoka nivasucu* is really a socially acceptable way for a woman to express her distress, and that distress, in turn, can only exist because her social milieu has failed her. In Fiji, *na tadoka nivasucu* has the effect of mobilizing social resources for new mothers (Becker 1998). In other words, to Fijians, *na tadoka nivasucu* represents not a malfunction in a woman's biology but rather a weakness in her social support system.

The Blues, Clinical Depression, and Psychosis

Now that we've begun to think about depression—its causes and who gets it—differently, let's make sure that we know exactly what we're talking about when we use the term depression and specifically what is and what is not postpartum depression.

In the introduction for this book, we took a look at the definition of depression. As you'll recall, the DSM currently describes depression as a major mood disorder that includes symptoms like feelings of hopelessness, insomnia or oversleeping, and increased pessimism. But the symptoms of what we commonly think of as PPD can be broken down into three categories: the "baby blues," clinical depression, and psychosis.

Even though the experiences are sometimes conflated, it's not at all clear that the baby blues, clinical depression, and postpartum psychosis are the same thing. These three things might very well be different entities unto themselves. What we call the blues is so common in Western culture and (was) so totally absent in other cultures (Nigeria, Japan, Fiji, Malaysia, and China, to name but a few) that I have to conclude, along with the anthropologists, that the blues is a culture-bound syndrome, a function of how Western culture experiences vulnerability and trains women to attend to and label physiological fluctuations in emotional terms (Harkness 1987; Stern and Kruckman 1983). To get more clarity, let's look at what each of these terms really means.

Baby blues. Some Western women experience tearfulness and emotional vulnerability when their milk comes in. They feel a little rattled, on edge, and weepy. This state has been characterized as the new-baby blues, and some think of it as clinical depression lite—different only in degree of severity. We've already seen that our major Internet sources of information about mental health attribute this emotional vulnerability to the drop in estrogen and progesterone that occurs after delivery. But is it, really?

You've just had a baby, for crying out loud. Why wouldn't you be emotional? How awesome is it to be in the delivery room and witness the miracle of life? Heck, every time I've watched a woman give birth I've been so awed, so deeply moved by the beauty of it all, that I've been more emotionally vulnerable for some time afterward. Why wouldn't dads feel moved, awed, and emotional? Why wouldn't adoptive parents feel emotional after their long-awaited hopes have finally come to fruition? Lottery winners do. The most normal response in the world to birth is awe, an overwhelming roller coaster of emotions. Not to mention that sleep deprivation by itself will increase emotional vulnerability (Kahn-Greene et al. 2006). The baby blues could realistically be thought of as simple emotional overwhelm mixed with awe, fear, and considerable fatigue.

Depression. *Clinical depression,* on the other hand, involves much more than emotional vulnerability and tearfulness. It tends to be considered as more severe than the baby blues, and it includes many or all of the symptoms mentioned in the DSM.

Clinical depression does seem to vary across different cultures, but only in terms of which symptoms are most salient—what aspects of experience are attended to and reported. So, while the most common and most troublesome symptoms for someone in Thailand, Paraguay, or Morocco might be slightly different from the symptoms that get reported most often in the United States, Canada, and England, symptoms of depression are symptoms of *depression,* nonetheless. Clinical depression is not the more quickly resolved tears and low energy of the baby blues.

Psychosis. Psychosis is an altogether different problem. *Postpartum psychosis,* an episode of mental illness involving a complete break with reality, is probably a variant of bipolar disorder or schizoaffective illness rather than a type of depression (Chaudron 2003; Nager, Johansson, and Sundquist 2006). But it's not at all clear, not at all uniform, and sometimes sheer exhaustion and sleep deprivation can trigger a psychotic episode in someone who would otherwise not be considered mentally ill (Sharma, Smith, and Khan 2004). In fact, postpartum psychosis has been documented in an adoptive mother: "A twenty-nine-year-old woman was hospitalized three weeks after adopting a full-term infant from an agency. She believed she was pregnant with the twin of her adopted child, whom she feared losing to the adoption agency. She had slept minimally, worrying that she might not hear her baby crying" (Van Putten and LaWall 1981, 1087). Postpartum psychosis has also been identified in fathers (Bucove 1964; Shapiro and Nass 1986; Van Putten and LaWall 1981).

These three phenomena are, on the surface, very similar in that they all involve sad or distressing emotions and can occur after childbirth. And all three are commonly understood as being part of what we think of as postpartum depression. But lumping these three separate experiences together under one label tends to equate them. Thus, tearing up and feeling blue is thought of in the same category as all-out psychosis—they're both postpartum depression. This conflation can serve to make *any* negative or vulnerable emotions a parent experiences after their baby is born seem extraordinarily scary and alarming. In our culture, where medical and legal concerns are often intertwined, incomplete understandings about emotions can lead to overreactions and to overmedicating normally occurring feelings.

Infanticide: Dispelling the Fears

"Infanticide" is a scary word, a term that brings up lots of horrifying thoughts and fears. Especially when you're feeling low, perhaps angry, and at the end of your rope, you may not want to even see the word in print, much less think about its meaning. But exploring the truth about this phenomenon and making sure you understand what it really is and how often it actually happens can go a long way toward easing your mind.

Many people associate postpartum psychosis with the story of Andrea Yates, the Texas mother who drowned all five of her children and was found not guilty by reason of insanity. Her diagnosis was postpartum psychosis because she was indeed psychotic, and she was six months postpartum. Yet there was a much larger and more complex context to her mental illness. This wasn't your "everyday" bout of postpartum psychosis, even if that's how much of the media presented it.

Andrea Yates had been depressed for a long time. She had several hospitalizations, not all of which were related to her pregnancies. She had been psychotic long before she drowned her children. Postpartum psychosis did not strike out of the clear blue; rather, it was part of her long and involved struggle with mental illness. According to news reports and court testimony, Andrea Yates had been suicidal and had told people that she was suicidal specifically because she was having urges to harm her children. Nor were her thoughts of harming her children the random musings of a troubled mind. In fact she was deeply involved in a fundamentalist religious cult, and her delusions centered around her belief that if she was not a *perfect* mother then her children would go to hell. So, rather than risk that, she felt it better to send them to heaven and take on the punishment of the legal system herself—a punishment she felt she deserved. Andrea Yates' psychosis framed her murders as loving acts of sacrifice. Her thinking clearly followed the lines of cognitive distortions that are characteristic of depression, but the magnitude of her distortions was so extreme as to constitute a break with reality, or psychosis (Roche 2002).

Andrea Yates apparently committed infanticide during one of the many psychotic episodes that she suffered after becoming completely desperate. She was overwhelmed on every front: by her role as mother, her oppressive religious beliefs, and a difficult relationship with a husband who did not know how to be supportive to her in the ways that would have been most helpful and meaningful. She is *not* representative of postpartum depression or of postpartum psychosis— or even of parents who commit infanticide.

The U.S. Department of Justice defines *infanticide* as the murder of any child under the age of five (Federal Bureau of Investigation 2004). According to this definition, there were 18,711 cases of infanticide in the U.S. between 1976 and 2005. This averages out to about 624 per year. Of these, 31 percent were committed by fathers, 29 percent were committed by mothers, and 23 percent were committed by a male acquaintance. Clearly, with a U.S. population of 304 million, these figures are minute.

Distinguishing Fantasy from Danger

While infanticide remains incredibly rare, fantasizing about harming an infant, in contrast, is very common. According to a study done by Susan Levitski and Robyn Cooper in 2000, 70 percent of mothers of colicky infants acknowledged having had thoughts of harming their child when they were difficult to soothe and 26 percent actually thought about infanticide. But *none* of these women acted on their fantasies or even felt that they were in serious danger of doing so. And that, too, is an important point. Andrea Yates not only had the fantasies, she also had the urges; she not only had the urges, she lacked impulse control. Andrea Yates knew she was not able to safely contain her urges, and she told people around her so.

Thoughts are thoughts; actions are actions. Not all thoughts lead to actions. Not all feelings lead to actions. Most people, even depressed people, do *not* kill their children. Most people do not kill their children even when they have vivid fantasies of doing something, *anything,* to stop the annoying demands of a difficult-to-soothe infant. Yet, many women who struggle with postpartum depression feel afraid that psychosis might "strike" them, and that they will then do the "unthinkable"—even though they are not psychotic, do not have irresistible urges to harm their children, and are probably not really at risk for committing murder. Popular books on postpartum depression, unclear about the research and what it means, fuel these fears. They create unnecessary guilt and fear and exacerbate treatable depression. Such fears, in turn, add layers of emotional distance between the mother and her new baby, which can be unnecessarily damaging to both.

In reality, postpartum depression is clinical depression, plain and simple. It is not qualitatively different from major depression diagnosed at any other point in the life cycle, and it doesn't affect only women (as we've seen). Rather, the word postpartum is merely an adjective used as additional diagnostic information describing the timing of the onset or occurrence of the clinically diagnosable depressive episode. Clinical depression, any clinical depression, *is* potentially dangerous, as suicide is a real risk. While this book will help you start the process of feeling better and assist you in staying on that road, if you have been diagnosed with clinical depression, it's best to also get help from a qualified and competent licensed mental health professional.

Depression Is Increasing Worldwide

According to the World Health Organization, depression is a leading cause of human suffering worldwide and has been steadily increasing over the past several decades (World Health Organization 1999). When looking at diseases and disorders, epidemiologists study *morbidity*, meaning the ways that diseases destroy and diminish lives, as well as *mortality*, meaning how often and how these ailments result in death. They use statistical means to estimate YLDs, which are "years lived with disability," and DALYs, or "disability-adjusted life years." *Disability-adjusted life years* are understood as the sum of years of potential life lost due to premature mortality and the years of productive life lost due to disability. Depression is already the second leading cause of DALYs among fifteen- to forty-four-year-olds of either sex, worldwide, and by 2020, the World Health Organization projects that depression will be the second leading cause of DALYs for *all* ages and both sexes worldwide. Postpartum depression has also been on the rise, afflicting cultures where it was once unheard of and unknown (Becker and Lee 2002).

What About Blue Genes?

But what causes depression, and why is it on the rise? It has long been assumed that there must be biological markers for the tendency to become depressed, and these markers must surely have a genetic basis. After all, we know that depression does tend to run in families.

When the human genome project came out, people jumped on it, looking for evidence that there must be one gene for every illness. Some researchers referred rather tongue-in-cheek to this as the "O, GOD" hypothesis—O, GOD being an acronym for "one gene; one disease." Very few diseases have turned out to have one gene as their cause. And mental illnesses have completely failed to show any such simplistic patterns.

When I was in graduate school many years ago, the dominant paradigm that was taught was called the *diathesis stress* model. This model assumes that people respond to stress differently depending on their genetic makeup, and so stress results in different problems for different people. Some people develop ulcers under stress and, it was assumed, some people develop depression. But now it looks like this model might need to be qualified and refined—the truth is more nuanced and perhaps even more malleable.

To explore what genetics may have to do with mental health, the National Institutes of Health convened a panel of distinguished scientists from many different disciplines, all relevant to the study of the genetics of mood disorders. The panel included researchers in molecular biology, population genetics, statistical genetics, genetic epidemiology, behavioral genetics, adult and child psychiatry, and developmental psychology. This panel was charged with developing a strategic plan for employing the tools of genetics to advance the understanding and treatment of mood disorders in hopes of improving the outcome of mood disorders (depression, anxiety disorders, and the bipolar spectrum). In 2002, the panel published their results (Merikangas et al. 2002).

Noting that while there is some possibility that a gene link to bipolar and anxiety disorders may eventually be found, there is much less promise of the eventual discovery of a genetic link when it comes to simple depression. The panel recommended that instead of looking for a single gene for depression, research should focus rather on identifying the genetic markers for the kinds of vulnerabilities that might give rise to depression in the *context* of stressful life changes. This would have implications for postpartum depression because having a baby is a hugely stressful major life change, and we need to know if a resulting depression is really inescapable. The vulnerabilities that are most likely to have some genetic component are what are referred to as "core components" of mood disorders—mood regulation, autonomic reactivity (that part of your nervous system that is set to detect and respond to emotionally loaded material), sleep regulation, and stress responsivity (Merikangas et al. 2002). These core components are temperamental variables that occur in different measures in different people. *Temperament* is the raw material of personality that a child is born with. The more experience you have around babies, the clearer it is that babies react differently to bright lights, loud sounds, strong smells, and so forth. Some babies are easy to handle and other babies seem to protest more when they are handled or when their environment changes. These are the basics, the wet clay, so to speak, of what later becomes personality. And these temperamental variables (that have to do with how reactive the nervous system is) are what seem to be the basis of heritable vulnerabilities to depression.

But even these vulnerabilities interact with learning and environment, so that many people who have these genetic vulnerabilities never actually go on to develop depression. This NIH panel of distinguished scientists also predicted that recurrent depression, particularly when it starts in childhood, will probably turn out to be a manifestation of bipolar disorder. But the jury is still out, and we won't know for sure until we have a lot more research to go on.

Several of these same researchers recently authored a paper that appeared in the July 2009 issue of the *Journal of the American Medical Association (JAMA)*. This paper detailed a meta-analysis of all the available genetic studies on depression. Since medications known as serotonin selective reuptake inhibitors, or SSRIs, are the most popular drugs used to treat depression, the neurochemistry of serotonin is what is most studied. As a specific gene for serotonin transport has been discovered, the researchers assumed that the serotonin-transporter gene is the one that is most likely to be behind depression—that is, *if* depression has a single genetic cause.

The results were surprising. The researchers concluded, "This meta-analysis yielded no evidence that the serotonin-transporter genotype alone *or in interaction with stressful life events* [italics added] is associated with an elevated risk of depression in men alone, women alone, or in both sexes combined" (Risch et al. 2009). Wow. Not only was there absolutely no relationship between the serotonin-transporter gene and depression, there was no relationship between the serotonin-transporter gene, stress, and depression. In other words, the so-called depression gene isn't even activated by stress to cause depression (Risch et al. 2009). So, whatever genetic contributions might be involved in creating a vulnerability to depression, they're clearly not simple, not a matter of a single gene, and probably set in motion by many other environmental factors.

If Not Genes, What Does Cause Depression?

If there isn't a single gene for depression, or even a gene that results in depression when activated by stress, then what does cause depression? Psychologists, who are not medical doctors, have long taken a very different (and nonmedical) approach to research in mental illness. And psychological research has consistently pointed out that depressed people have a very particular way of looking at life—an attributional style (Abramson, Seligman, and Teasdale 1978; Abramson, Metalsky, and Alloy 1989).

Attributions are ways of looking at life, especially ways of thinking about the bad things that happen, and I'll be explaining them further in the next chapter. Besides having a particular way of looking at life (these and other unhelpful habits of thought are commonly thought of as *cognitive vulnerabilities*), depressed people also have a particular way of relating to others, which can be thought of as *interpersonal vulnerabilities* (Katz and Joiner 2001; Pettit and Joiner 2006b; Potthoff, Holahan, and Joiner 1995). It turns out that depressed people tend to relate to others in ways that elicit rejection and thereby put themselves at risk for depression (Joiner 1995). In chapter 3 we'll look at those habits of relating, the interpersonal risk factors, or what we might call the "social side" of depression.

Depression clearly also has biological aspects—sleep and appetite disturbance, decreased or absent sex drive, an inability to experience pleasure—aspects that I don't want to gloss over or dismiss in any way. But it's not at all clear that biological events *cause* depression, while it *is* quite clear that nonbiological variables, things like habits of thought and patterns of relating, can change biology. This reciprocal and dynamic action between thoughts, feelings, and biology will be a theme throughout this book. Though it may not seem as simple as a magic bullet (take a pill, feel better), it's important to take the time to understand that emotions are complex, circular bio-psycho-social events. When we understand how and why emotions arise and linger, then we can learn to change and manage them.

Exercises for Chapter 1

At the end of each chapter in *After the Stork*, I'll be offering exercises. These simple tasks will help you integrate the new material you're learning and will assist you in keeping track of and sorting through your thoughts and experiences. I encourage you to get a notebook and pencil, to try the exercises, jotting down your thoughts and observations.

Exercise 1: Create a Vision

This first exercise will help you cast your mind toward better times, when you feel better and your life is more comfortable. Allow yourself to fantasize about how you'd like your life to be when it's better. Instead of imagining a problem-free life, imagine a life where you feel happy and in control of your emotions, able to face and solve your problems day in and day out with equanimity.

For instance, imagine waking up with the baby and feeling okay about it. You're not as tired. You don't feel anxious or stressed or hopeless. You feel good about seeing your little one and being able to spend time with him or her. You know you can handle what comes your way. Now imagine one or two other scenes that represent your new life as you'd like it to be. You can choose feeding the baby, being with your partner, going out with the baby, anything that appeals to you. Now describe your vision in your notebook.

Now go back and examine how you see yourself interacting with your baby and your partner (if you have one) in this fantasy. Describe how you *feel* and how you *interact* in detail. In your notebook, write down what you discover.

Exercise 2: Name Your Fears

Go ahead and take a moment to write down your greatest fears about becoming a parent. This may seem challenging at first. Please remember that writing down a fear doesn't make it more real. In fact, it's often a relief to see a fear in black and white. That way, you can see how unrealistic or unlikely it is. But even if your fears seem just as real to you after writing them down, try to remember that bringing them to light and working with them is a great way of working *through* them, much like turning on the light and looking under the bed, if you were afraid of "the monster under your bed" when you were a kid. Doing this work is a positive step toward feeling better.

Keep your list relatively short for starters—say about five items. Write each item on a different page of a notebook, one page per fear, and keep your notebook close at hand at all times. Some people like to use a small notebook that will fit into a purse, and others carry a large diaper bag and so prefer a larger notebook. Just try to be sure your notebook is handy.

Now challenge yourself to notice reassuring evidence and the reassuring words you might get each day. When we're in the grip of fear, we often disregard or even fail to notice evidence contrary to our fears. Instead, I'd like you to pay special attention to more positive evidence and write it down under the fear it counters. Some examples for items of evidence you might notice are:

* Supportive comments from people around you

* An instance when something you feared not only didn't happen, but instead actually went well

* A good feeling you weren't expecting to have

* Times when something bad or undesirable happened but you coped

Don't be stingy with your evidence. Write down everything you notice that can be understood as countering your fear. One of the things that reliably gets people into trouble is that they ask terrible, horrible, "what if" questions about unlikely events and keep going round and round in their mind about these worst-case scenarios. So if you're going to ask yourself a "what if," then you have to go ahead and answer it. And the answer is always some variant of "it would suck but I would deal." Tormenting yourself with "what if" questions is really about trying to control the future and how much distress you have to deal with in life—and neither of those things is really under your control. If something bad happens it will suck and you will deal. Meanwhile, there's so much to enjoy about life if you turn your mind and just settle into what is. Another thing that ties people in knots is that they don't really know how to assess the probabilities—so they are afraid of flying on an airplane, for example, but they drive a car every day. What are the probabilities of someday having a car wreck as compared to someday being in an airplane accident? And even if they do assess probabilities correctly, they overlook the basic fact that probabilities predict for the population, not for the individual. In other words, there are no guarantees in life. You do the best you can and you have to get comfortable with the everyday risks that go with life.

Exercise 3: Set Learning Goals

For those things that you're genuinely not good at, for those frustrating qualities in yourself that you wish were different, set learning goals. Learning goals have to be very *specific* and very *stair-stepped*. In other words, break each goal down into small, bite-sized pieces that are clearly defined. Learning proceeds through attention to evidence of progress, so pay attention to your successes. Embrace the learning curve. Talk to other people who have undertaken difficult learning curves. What kept them going in the face of discouragement?

So, doing this exercise means:

1. Coming up with goals for learning that are important to you

2. Putting them in order according to priority

3. Breaking each goal down into workable steps

4. Noting and celebrating when you accomplish each of the steps

5. Writing each phase in your notebook

This exercise is important because it will help you take a longer view (which is sometimes difficult when you are depressed) and will provide a framework that will get you moving. Small steps are key, as is really giving yourself credit for your achievements. Think about each step as a new opportunity to give yourself a pat on the back.

One of my clients recently told me about her son and her daughter. Her son has what she called low self-esteem and doesn't want to try anything hard. Her daughter doesn't seem to have this problem. Her daughter asked to learn to roller skate when she was five. She had a blast learning, and now she can do all sorts of wheelies and has promoted herself to inline skates. Once she got really good at inline skating, she asked her mother if she could have ice-skating lessons. My client's son, in contrast, keeps picking goals that are star quality. You can't get to be the best if you're not willing to start at the bottom. Figure out what's fun about learning and keep raising the bar little by little.

Exercise 4:
Cultivating Appreciation

Notice what you take for granted. How long have you lived in your neighborhood? How many times have you walked the same three blocks? Given how naturally the human mind works, it's almost guaranteed that you don't know what you haven't noticed. So here's some homework to try. Grab your notebook and take a walk around your neighborhood with a specific task in mind: to notice ten things you've never noticed before. How many times have you walked past the Murphys' without noticing that they have a birdfeeder in the back yard? Have you ever noticed how the light changes in the kitchen over the course of the day? Keep going ... I'll bet you can't stop at just ten.

CHAPTER 2

Habits of Thought

Such as are your habitual thoughts, such also will be the character of your mind; for the soul is dyed by the thoughts.

Marcus Aurelius Antoninus

Like so many middle-class couples these days, Lou and Casey planned their first child. They worried a little bit when it took them longer than expected to get pregnant, but when it finally happened they were ecstatic. The months of pregnancy went by uneventfully for the most part, with doctors' visits, encouraging friends, and doting relatives marveling at Lou's growing belly and the inevitable deluge of baby showers when her due date drew near. No one expected Lou to collapse in a puddle once she got home with the baby, but collapse she did. And no one was more surprised than Lou—unless maybe it was Casey. Lou said that she felt like she was down at the bottom of a well trying to look up but not seeing any light. Casey was horrified to see how little interest she showed in the baby. Even Lou's mother was alarmed and took turns with her sisters staying over so Lou and Casey could get a full night's sleep.

Lou looked like something the cat dragged in—she had deep circles under her eyes, which were red from crying. She was so horrified at her own reaction to the baby that she thought everyone would be better off without her. She wanted to run away, but she had nowhere to run to.

She wanted to die, but thankfully, her faith prevented her from taking any action to end her own life. Every time the baby cried she cringed and recoiled; then, noticing her own reaction, she wept. "I'm a terrible mother," she moaned. "My baby deserves better." Avoiding holding or talking to her infant seemed like an act of self-sacrifice and honorable giving. "It's better that someone else hold her—I'm no good at this," she would say. Later, when she felt better, Lou described this time of her life as "living in a cartoon." She felt as if she was observing life, not participating in it. Try as she might, she couldn't bridge the gap on her own. Everything seemed to be playing out in slow motion, strangely disconnected from feeling.

Like Lou, not everyone falls in love with their baby at first sight, but just about everyone I meet expected to. Parenting skills do not necessarily rise up out of the soul complete with a deep conviction of competence—many first-time parents will necessarily find themselves at the bottom of a learning curve. Most new parents have some idea that sleep deprivation comes with the territory, but knowing about something is often quite different from experiencing it. Coping with the fatigue of sleeplessness is not for the fainthearted. Lou was a labor and delivery nurse. She had coached many women through labor and watched wistfully as they left the hospital with bundles in their arms. She was a confident professional and quite competent at her job. But she didn't know the first thing about mothering—she was going to have to let the baby teach her that part. And she hated feeling stupid. So when she wasn't filled with joyous motherly feelings she judged herself harshly, attributing her lack of competence and disappointing lack of positive emotions to a deep, immutable, core defect in herself.

Culture Shapes Thoughts, and Thoughts Shape Reality

Psychologists used to think that all people think the same way, attending to the same cues to make sense of the world. But new research shows that habits of thought are very much shaped by culture and expectations (Goode 2000; Nisbett and Masuda 2007; Masuda and

Nisbett 2001). Habits of thought are learned and transmitted socially in the family and the culture.

The key to a habit is in the repetition. Once established, a habit tends to be unconscious and automatic. How we think, the strategies we use to decide what information is relevant and worth attending to, and the strategies we use to process information that we have extracted from the world around us are also habits—repeated often enough to become automatic and largely unconscious. And habits of thought generate emotions, including depression.

This may seem unlikely, because emotions seem like the opposite of thought: as one psychologist put it, "the laws of emotion are grounded in mechanisms that are not of a voluntary nature and that are only partially under voluntary control" (Frijda 1988, 349). But while emotions themselves are not voluntary, the *meanings* that give rise to emotions are thoughts, and thoughts *are* under voluntary control. The first "law" of emotions is that they result from the meanings we assign to events. (Frijda 1988, 349). In other words, meanings are thoughts.

Psychologists have been researching the relationship between how people think, what people do, and whether depression results for many decades. Several key variables have consistently emerged and have been repeatedly confirmed. People who are prone to depression have a particular cognitive style that predisposes them to become depressed whenever stressful events accumulate in their lives (Beck and Alford 2009; Ciesla and Roberts 2007; Beck 2005). And *cognitive style* is just a fancy way to say habits of thought. In other words, people who are prone to depression—people who become depressed—have predictable patterns to their habits of thought that reliably lead to depression.

This also means that "emotions change when meanings change ... when events are viewed differently" (Frijda 1988, 350). You do have some way to control your emotions and your emotional experiences. So the key to preventing and overcoming depression rests on first cultivating awareness of automatic habits of thought and then deliberately changing the habits of thought that lead to depression (Fava et al. 1998; Burns and Nolen-Hoeksema 1991; Frijda 1988).

Lou was in the habit of holding herself to high standards. She was used to feeling competent and knowledgeable, so she felt she should know things about mothering that she really had no way of knowing.

She habitually took charge and did what needed to be done. But faced with a new situation, she wasn't able to be flexible or patient with herself or gentle with her own learning curve. In this chapter, we'll be looking closely at three major habits of thought that make us vulnerable to depression. Different researchers slice the pie differently, and there are many different ways to look at habits of thought. I've chosen the ones that are interrelated and that I find most commonly in my practice.

Cognitive Risk Factors for Depression

There are actually five common habits of thought that tend to make my clients vulnerable to depression. However, they tend to overlap, and some only appear aligned with others. Within the chapter as a whole, I'll be framing the discussion by focusing on the three primary habits; but, to begin with, I'll offer a brief definition of all five. They are:

- **Global Thinking:** Overly inclusive, black-and-white thinking that overlooks nuance and context

- **External Locus of Control:** The sense that the source of distress is outside of oneself

- **Tendency to Internalize Blame:** Often feeling responsible for things that are not under your control and, therefore, feeling blameworthy

- **Personalized Rejection:** A tendency to feel hyper-alert to cues indicating possible rejection and to feel that being rejected must be your fault

- **Discomfort with Uncertainty:** Difficulty getting comfortable with the uncertainties of everyday life; having trouble with self-soothing

These habits tend to work together, one influencing and promoting another, to produce an increased vulnerability to depression. Now let's take a closer look at each one.

Global, Binary Thinking

If you have a global cognitive style, it means that you tend to see the forest and not the individual trees—the big picture always pops into view first, which can easily become overwhelming. It is easy to read one chapter in a book, but it's much harder to read one chapter if you're thinking about how many chapters you have to read over how many years in order to earn a degree. Overly global thinkers are usually not very nuanced in their thinking. Because they see the big picture easily and the details with difficulty, they tend to quickly divide the world into black and white, good and bad, right and wrong, true and false, us and them, and so on, without taking context into account (Yapko 1997). And context can make all the difference in the world. I call this style *binary thinking*.

So when Lou came home from the hospital with a baby, and she didn't instantly feel a flood of love, affection, and familiarity with this little person, binary thinking led her to conclude that she's a "bad mom." As if there are only two kinds of moms in the world—good ones and bad ones—and she is all bad. A new dad who notices that his best friend, his wife, now has little time for him, or who feels annoyed with the baby's crying, might conclude that he is not cut out for fatherhood. The same person who, just a few days ago, *was* a good wife, a good friend, or a good person is now abruptly a bad mother or bad father—and that's it. No nuance, no room for shades of gray. You can see how thinking of yourself as simply bad could make you feel pretty lousy.

Binary Thinking and the Quest for Perfection

Binary thinkers generally work very hard to be perfect because the smallest evidence of failure, disappointment, or human frailty will easily flip them into thinking they are bad instead of good, and thinking "I am bad" feels terrible. Global thinkers also tend to be concrete—to trust what they can see, feel, taste, touch, and hear in the immediate present. More abstract concepts are harder for them to work with. So, if they aren't facing tangible evidence that they are what they consider a good person in the immediate moment, they are vulnerable to a binary flip. If they have no evidence that they're good, they must be bad. As you can imagine, they work very hard to keep evidence of their goodness in front of them, but that sneaky, sneaky, evidence to the contrary is always close at hand—we humans are, after all, inevitably flawed. And that's exactly what Lou did. She went from noticing that this being a parent gig was all new, to concluding that she was a defective human being.

Binary thinkers tend to think in terms of always and never. So, if they feel irrational feelings of irritation toward a completely innocent baby right this minute, then not only is that evidence that they are bad instead of good, but they often imagine that this feeling will last forever and is a *permanent* quality of their core selves. Global thinkers generate permanent, pervasive, and personal attributions (or explanations) for negative events (Seligman 1990). In other words, a global thinker, like Lou, is apt to read a situation that feels negative as proving that she will *always* behave or feel a certain way, that this indicates something about her essential self that will never change.

Take a look at Lou's attributions: "I'm a terrible mother" was a permanent attribution instead of a contextual one (for instance, "I'm having a hard time with mothering right now, in these circumstances"). Thinking of herself as a terrible mother was deeply personal and presupposed permanence. When she thought, "My baby deserves better," she assumed that her inadequacies were permanent, personal, and pervasive. "I'm no good at this" suggested that she and she alone was defective, immutable, and unteachable. She felt to blame for something that she had little control over, as if parenting skills were "out there" instead of "in here," resident inside of her in rough form, like a lump of clay waiting to be shaped. She was the potter, but she was looking around outside of herself for someone to shape those skills for her. How different she felt later when she was able to laugh at herself lovingly, expecting and accepting that the learning curve may be steep and slow to climb. How different she felt when she finally realized that the baby didn't know how to be a baby any more than she knew how to be a mother or Casey knew how to be a daddy. By allowing this possibility, Lou began to see that she could shape the baby, the baby could shape her, and together they would become family.

Sam, another of my clients, just had her fourth child; it was her husband's first. She refers to him as a "beginner parent" and laughs at how much his anxiety and his learning curve resemble her first experience as a parent. Sam, like most experienced parents, has learned to take herself much less seriously than she once did. By doing so, she also takes herself off the hook of having to be perfect.

Emotional Intensity

One of the things we know about emotions from more than forty years of science and research is that a global cognitive style makes emotions feel more intense. And, it's also true that whenever emotions become intense—whether the intensity comes from the cognitive style applied to an accumulation of negative events over time (as when a series of changes coincide in a person's life) or whether the intensity comes from a temperamental predisposition to experience emotions more vividly, emotional intensity constricts cognitive processing. What does this mean? Well, as emotions intensify, cognitive processes (including attention, concentration, and memory) constrict. It is as though emotions and thoughts are related in a closed system, like a balloon or piece of clay—when you stretch the balloon or clay in one direction, it has to take up slack from the other because there is just so much air or clay available. And when emotions become intense, the biological tendency of the organism, whether human or animal, is to conserve resources. While this system may be efficient in the wild, it causes problems in our complex, postmodern world because it means we lose the nuances that come with taking a variety of contextual information into account (Frijda 1988; Linehan 1993b).

Locus of Control

People who are prone to depression often also tend to have an *external locus of control* in addition to a global cognitive style. This means that when something distressing happens, they conclude that it's being inflicted on them by something outside of themselves; that they have no control over the situation.

Lou felt completely out of control. She didn't know what to do when the baby cried, so she would try different things. But when the first one or two things she tried failed, she was left bewildered. Lou felt that she was responsible for keeping the baby happy at all times; she couldn't distinguish between what she was responsible for and what she was *not* responsible for. So, besides feeling like the source of her distress was outside of herself, she felt to blame. And Lou's ways of thinking are typical of people struggling with depression. What a catch-22—you have no control over events, but you're responsible for them. It is as if the cause of emotions is in the environment, but you are responsible for controlling your environment, which is often unresponsive to your efforts.

For instance, an infant cries for many different reasons. But if you have an external locus of control and you internalize blame, you will be more likely to feel that the situation is outside of your control (which may very well be true, if the baby is difficult to soothe). The real kicker is that you tend to use that fact—that the baby is crying and you can't control her—as evidence of your inadequacy. This dynamic of externalizing control while internalizing blame means that you feel you must control your external environment in order to be comfortable in your own skin. And, because it's impossible to totally control your environment (especially with an infant in the house), you inevitably feel like a failure. Lou, like many new parents, was caught up in just this kind of pattern. Phew ... what a tiresome circle!

A Tendency to Internalize Blame

Being able to take responsibility is a good thing. But the tendency can go awry and cause a lot of unnecessary emotional distress if you are making yourself responsible for things that you have little or no influence over. The ability to accurately distinguish where your influence (and therefore responsibility) ends and external forces take over is essential for mental health.

A Habit of Personalizing Rejection

Our lives are inexorably intertwined with others, and so my choices impact others and others' choices impact me. Sometimes I'm distracted, or in a hurry, or moody. My words or actions might not measure up to what another person expects of me. The same goes for everyone else. If I hold too tightly to my expectations and interpret other people's behavior as rejection, sometimes I might be right—but a lot of times I'm bound to be wrong. Being able to accurately attribute someone else's behavior, behavior that I find disappointing, to the situation, their personality, or social signaling is essential to my own happiness and to my ability to navigate complex social situations. So, if I know that I'm sensitive to rejection, I might need to develop compensatory strategies for getting accurate information—my feelings will not be a very good compass in many social contexts.

I think of this skill set as falling under the category of boundaries. Having good boundaries means that you know where you end and someone else begins, and it therefore means that you take good care of yourself. Holding your boundaries means you let your yes be yes and your no be no, confident that you can manage your own disappointments and other people can manage theirs.

Categories and Criteria

It is important to have categories and criteria—flexible ways of organizing information and clear criteria for knowing when one rule applies and when a different rule applies. If I have flexible categories (instead of binary ones) then I can take in more information and consider the context before I reach conclusions. But people like Lou, who are prone to depression and who have a global cognitive style, also often don't know how to decide which rule to apply in what context. They lack clarity about what level of analysis to apply—what level of categories and what kinds of criteria. Even experienced parents like Sam have to figure out *this* baby—meaning they embark on a learning curve to decipher the *specific* meaning of *this* baby's cues and preferences. If you listen to the conversations of people who have several children, you'll likely hear them comment on *how* their children were alike and *how* they were different. They are telling you about how they learned to categorize their experiences with each child and the criteria they developed in the process—the things they learned from the experience in parenting different children.

Lacking categories of context and sorting criteria renders life overwhelming, the smallest decisions exhausting (Yapko 1997). In a now-famous study published in 1958, scientist Joseph Brady trained monkeys to distinguish between circles and squares. He then began punishing them for errors in sorting (using a mild shock), while at the same time making the squares look more and more like circles so that the task was harder. Eventually the circles and squares were virtually indistinguishable and the shocks therefore inevitable. The more ambiguous the task, the more the monkeys experienced anxiety, and the more likely they were to develop ulcers. Brady also yoked one monkey (which he called the "executive monkey") to another. In this variation of the experiment, the executive monkey had control while the yoked monkey did not. All the executive monkeys died of ulcers, but the yoked monkeys lived. This result led Brady to conclude that having control is more stressful than being the passive victim of painful experiences that one isn't in control of (Brady 1958). Even though it's a bit of a stretch to go from monkey ulcers to postpartum depression, the priciple applies—it's better for your health to let go of the idea that you have total control over your baby's happiness and comfort.

Learning Curves

Since babies come preformatted but without instructions, it necessarily means that parents learn sorting strategies through trial and error, a process that necessarily involves ambiguity—not knowing. Trial-and-error learning also needs to involve failure and frustration. Learning curves *always* involve some failure. But Lou, like many adults, was used to feeling competent, and she interpreted the necessary failures and frustrations of learning to parent as "screwups" and felt stupid about them. Her interpretation of the situation, of the learning curve, was the problem, *not* the fact that she didn't know what she was doing.

But people who have an external locus of control tend to want to control their environment in order to reduce their stress instead of looking for ways to change how they think about the events in their life. One reason for this can be the global cognitive style getting in the way yet again—if distressing emotions are caused by how I think, then it's my fault and I must be bad. But if distressing emotions are caused by something amiss in the environment, then perhaps I can succeed by trying harder. Lou was used to working hard; she wasn't used to thinking about how her thoughts give rise to emotions. She thought: "I am responsible for controlling the environment, and as long as I do that, I'm not bad; I'm in control. But the moment that I fail to control the environment, then I am bad."

Think about this setup for a moment. How much would it drive you crazy to live believing that you are either a "good" person *or* a "bad" person (with no shades of gray)? How painful is it to deeply (and often unconsciously) believe that nothing is truly under your control because everything is caused by some external agent, and yet you are to blame for everything that goes wrong (making you a bad person)? Wow. Sounds like a formula for depression. Actually, it is.

Internal Focus

Global thinkers who have an *external* locus of control blame themselves for everything unless they can find an external cause that lets them off the hook (Yapko 2001b). But oddly enough, these same people tend to look *inside* themselves for evidence about what is true—*cause* is outside, in the *environment,* but *truth* is *internal,* in feelings. In other words, they will look to their feelings to find out, for example, whether someone else is trustworthy. Lou looked inside herself, to her feelings, to find out if she was competent. She wasn't—yet. She looked inside herself, to her feelings, to find out if she was a good mother. But she failed to find the gushy warm emotions that she expected to constitute "love." This is what I mean by an internal focus. Locus of control is one thing and focus is another. Trusting *internal* feelings to tell you the truth about something *outside* of yourself is not very reliable and won't lead to very good choices.

New behaviors require learning. When you first start to learn something new, you don't even know how much you don't know, and that's the first stage of a learning curve. Then it dawns on you just how much there is to learn that you don't know yet, and that's the second stage of a learning curve. Then comes a time when you know more than you think you know, but you don't realize it yet—the third stage of a learning curve. Last comes the stage where you know what you need to know and you know that you know, and that *last* stage is when you have confidence, not before. Being unclear about what *is* about *you* and what is *not* about *you*, being unclear about what is under your control and what is not under your control, being unclear about what kind of information you need in what situations, is very bewildering.

So, to go back to the example of determining trustworthiness, wouldn't it be better to think in degrees? Instead of thinking about whether someone or something is or is not trustworthy, wouldn't it be better to think in terms of strengths and weaknesses in different contexts? If I expand my category of trustworthiness to include gradations and contexts, then I might begin to notice different things about people. I notice that Joan is overcommitted and has trouble saying no to reasonable requests. Therefore, I choose carefully what favors I ask of her and I always preface my requests with face-saving ways for her to decline. I notice that Susan is sometimes brusque and some people think her harsh. But I've also seen that she takes good care of herself and so I know I can trust her to tell me the truth when I ask for a favor. I notice that Patrick is great fun at a party and has very good social skills but often has trouble following through on promises and sometimes cuts corners on details. So, I invite Patrick to my parties but I don't count on him to check the details on a project we're working on together.

Tolerating Ambiguity

People who remain healthy and happy through life's ups and downs generally have well developed categories for parsing experience and clear criteria for distinguishing between what they *do* and *do not* have control over, and once they identify what they cannot control, they have good skills for making themselves comfortable with not knowing what is coming next. People like Lou, who are prone to depression, in contrast, often feel very confused about what is and is not under their control and expend large amounts of effort in trying to control elements of their world—things, events, and people. And when they fail, like Lou, they blame themselves. And since they have trouble sorting out what is and is not under their control, they typically don't have very well developed skills for tolerating ambiguity—letting go and getting comfortable with not knowing. Lou wanted clear-cut answers; she wanted her efforts to produce reliable results—a happy Gerber baby. Parenting a new baby is filled with ambiguity, so, as we will see in chapter 6, developing categories and criteria, along with strategies for getting comfortable with not knowing, are especially important skills.

Cognitive Styles and the Brain

We live in a culture where global thinking is very common and where most people make binary distinctions about what is "biological" and what is "mental." But this binary distinction is entirely false because every single thought that you have is biological. All thoughts are bio-chemical events that happen in your brain. So, if you can manage your thoughts, then you can manage the biochemistry of your brain. Let's take a closer look.

You may have seen pictures of what a brain looks like when it's outside the bony case we call the skull—all wrinkles and folds like some kind of spongy cloth wadded up to fit into a tight space. The tissues of the brain are made up of nerve cells called *neurons*. The neurons manufacture and contain chemicals called *neurotransmitters*. One neuron makes a connection with another neuron by releasing a neurotransmitter into the gap between them (this gap is called a *synapse*) (Banks 2001). Negative thoughts involve one class of neurotransmitter (broadly speaking, stress hormones) and positive thoughts involve another class of neurotransmitter (broadly speaking, endorphins). People who are global thinkers, who externalize control but internalize blame, and who have a bias toward negative thoughts, are going to generate more stress hormones than endorphins. Whenever something changes in their world, whenever they experience a disappointment, whenever they are uncertain or things that are very important to them are outside of their control, and when negative thoughts predominate over time, a chemical imbalance follows. Whatever neural connections are most often used, most practiced, most rehearsed, are going to be most automatic and stable. This is one reason why it is so important to become aware of your thoughts and begin to intentionally cultivate healthy habits of clear thinking and positivity.

The Biology of Emotions

Emotions come from thoughts. Emotions are also chemical events that start in the brain (Critchley 2009). But emotions are very complex events that occur in the body as well as in the brain (Linehan 1993a; Linehan 1993b). For example, when I get angry, muscle groups in my body become tense. The signature that anger produces in my body will necessarily be similar to the signature it produces in others, because we are all human beings, after all. Harry Stack Sullivan, one of the early fathers of the field of psychology, once said "we are all much more alike than different, much more simply human than otherwise" (1955, 32) and this is certainly true when it comes to how we experience emotions in the body. But there are also particular ways that I might experience anger (or any other emotion) that might be slightly different from how others experience this emotion. For example, I might tense my shoulders when I get angry, while you might tense your jaw. Thus, our experience of emotions is in some ways universal and in some ways unique.

Anger and fear are part of the "fight-or-flight" system of prepared-ness that all animals have as part of their survival mechanism. The fight-or-flight response is shorthand for the autonomic nervous system, and the longhand version is actually "fight, flight, freeze, feeding, and reproductive behavior." Just as the tongue starts out with four basic tastes: sweet, sour, salty, and bitter, so too there are a limited number of basic emotions: fear, anger, sadness, and joy (although the research on emotions is much less sophisticated than we might wish and there are differences of opinion about how many basic emotions there really are). All the nuances of taste, from garlic to chocolate ganache, all the wines, all the coffees, are given their subtleties by the combination of smell with these basic tastes. Similarly, emotions are given their subtle-ties when thoughts combine with basic emotions. And every emotion has an associated urge (Linehan 1993a; Linehan 1993b). Anger pairs with the urge to lash out. Fear pairs with the urge to flee. Sadness pairs with the urge to withdraw from others, from connection. Love pairs with the urge to connect and to bond. Each emotion is asso-ciated with a specific neurotransmitter or class of neurotransmitter (chemicals operating in the brain)—anger and fear with a variety of stress hormones like cortisol and adrenaline; sorrow with serotonin and the withdrawal of oxytocin; love, security, attachment, and satiation with endorphins like oxytocin, vasopressin, and dopamine (Frijda 1988). Science is a long way from understanding all the biochemical intricacies behind emotional experiencing, and human beings are not machines, so changing emotions and habits of thought will always have more in common with art than with science.

Culture, Chemicals, and Cognitive Style

Rather than there being a genetic predisposition or "chemical imbalance" that takes stressful life events and creates depression out of them, the set of symptoms we currently group together and label "depression" is more likely a set of learned habits of thought, habits of coping, and habits of relating that are learned in families and cultures. Of course our thoughts, emotions, and behavior are rooted in biology, and biologically, these are related to each other in particular ways. We have a natural tendency to narrow our thoughts when our emotions become intense, and this tendency can be more pronounced in some people than in others. How sensitive a person's nervous system is may be a function of temperament to some degree, but it can also be shaped by experience (Derryberry and Rothbart 1988; Banks 2001; Kagan, Reznick, and Snidman 1988).

Families and cultures, after all, are where we learn to interpret life, where we develop our cognitive style: whether we think in global, big-picture terms or more specifically (Kitayama et al. 2009; Freeman et al. 2009; Nisbett and Masuda 2007). Families and cultures are where we learn to attribute causes of things to external forces or develop many categories and criteria that allow us to attribute the causes of things to a more nuanced mix of factors that take context into account (Masuda and Nisbett 2001). Families and cultures are also where we learn to anticipate and defend against blame (Yapko 2009). Just as hormones aren't the only cause of postpartum depression, genes and biology aren't the only forces shaping emotions.

Social psychologists have repeatedly documented that culture shapes what people pay attention to. In a series of highly sophisticated experiments, researchers Richard Nisbett and Takahiko Masuda (2001) showed American and Japanese subjects a series of photographs and later quizzed them about what they had seen. Over and over again, the Japanese subjects remembered more details about the context of the pictures. Other researchers have shown that cultural differences not only shape perception but also carry over into attributions, so that East Asians, for example, are much more likely to take context into account when explaining the causes of other people's behavior (Peng and Nisbett 1999; Norenzayan, Choi, and Peng 2007). And these cultural differences in *what* is attended to and *how* meaning is construed is deeply rooted in the family. There is a fascinating field of research beginning to emerge about how parenting strategies are shaped by culture and, in turn, serve to pass on culture. Some of the findings are very subtle and surprising. In just one of many examples, researchers found that American parents correct their children directly, saying "no" or "that's wrong" and specifically pointing out the child's mistake or unacceptable behavior, while Japanese parents, in contrast, indirectly imply that the child made a mistake and then wait while the child attends to the context and infers his or her errors (Fernald and Morikawa 1993). This strategy teaches Japanese children to attend to multiple levels of meaning and many interpersonal cues and may be involved in shaping Japanese cultural values that emphasize group harmony over individuality. In contrast, our strategies may be part of how we perpetuate a more binary worldview.

Genes, Temperament, and Culture

Genes come into play in depression for only a small proportion of people (genetic factors at best account for about a third of the variance), and the contribution of genes to depression seems to mostly center around temperamental variables (Risch et al. 2009). Temperamental factors, like having a very sensitive nervous system that startles easily and is slow to soothe, could predispose a person to become emotionally reactive. An emotionally reactive temperament could poise a person to have fragile sleep. And having fragile sleep, could, when paired with the right habits of thoughts, predispose a person to slide more easily into depression than someone who sleeps well (Merikangas et al. 2002).

I have already touched on the vast literature that shows that culture shapes perception and cognition. But some scientists take this a step further and suggest that culture may itself be shaped, to some extent, by temperament and the genes behind temperament. For example, there is a large body of literature showing that Western European and East Asian babies consistently show temperamental differences (Kagan 2000). Western European infants tend to be more highly reactive than East Asian infants. Kagan (2000), citing several studies, writes:

> The most consistent set of data on early infant temperament compared Asian with Caucasian infants and found that the former were less reactive than the latter (Kagan et al. 1994). These ethnic differences in ease of becoming aroused might have derivatives in childhood. Chinese mothers of school-age children in Shanghai describe them as less active, less impulsive, and more controlled than mothers of Caucasian children living in the Pacific Northwest (Weisz et al. 1988). Moreover, Asian-American psychiatric patients require a lower dose of psychotropic drugs than do European-American patients with the same symptoms living in the same state. This fact implies that Asian populations may be at a lower level of limbic arousal (36).

Although it is highly speculative, it has been suggested that some of the differences in basic philosophies that shaped Eastern and Western thought may well be traceable in part to these temperamental differences, noting that Western Calvinism emphasizes anxiety, fear, and guilt, whereas Buddhist thought emphasizes calm, serenity, and detachment (Kagan, Arcus, and Snidman 1993).

How Thoughts Cause Depression

Now let's take a look at just how events, thoughts, emotions, and behaviors interact in depression. We'll start with some arbitrary starting point that I will call an "event." Old-school behaviorists might call it a "stimulus," and some people might call it the "trigger," but I just call it an event. The event that starts the sequence might be external or internal, something that happens to you, something someone else says or does, or something that you do, you say, or you think. Then—*zoop,*

zoop,—quicker than lightning, you have a feeling. The feeling invariably occurs in your body and involves an urge.

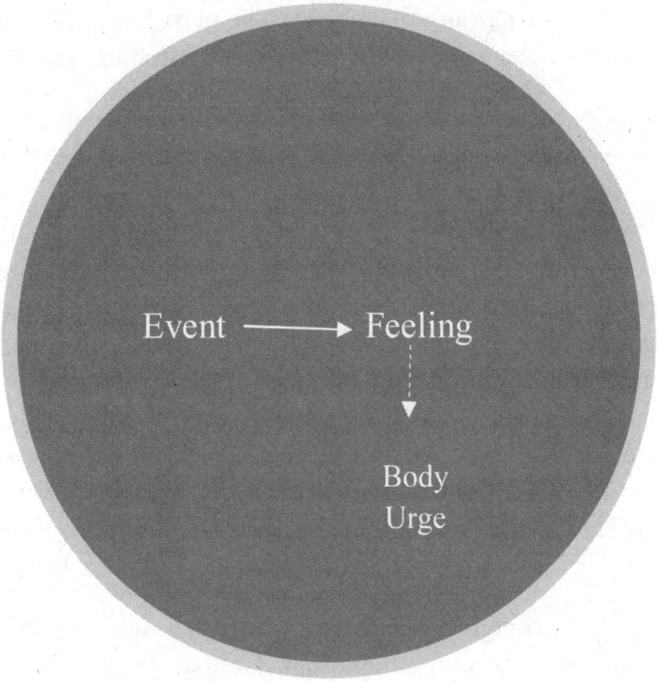

Event ⟶ Feeling

Body
Urge

Figure 2.1: Habits of Thought

In between the event and the feeling, often occurring just outside of awareness, is a thought process (Frijda 1988; Yapko 2009; Gross 1998). This thought process is your *interpretation* of the event, the meaning that you assign to it (Yapko 2009). This interpretation, this meaning, is necessarily colored by expectancies, which are based on past experiences, learned in family and culture, and inferred from context cues (Kirsch 1999). This process of interpretation and assigning meaning is largely automatic and unconscious, but it's this thought process that informs your brain's choice of feeling.

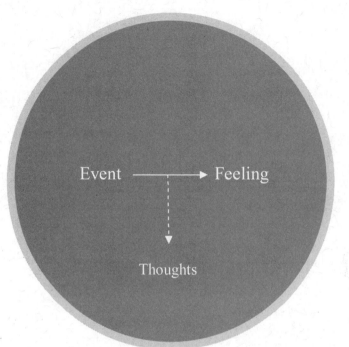

Figure 2.2: Habits of Thought

Then—*zoop, zoop,*—quicker than lightning again, you have a response. Your response might be internal, as when your heart drops when you hear bad news or your pulse quickens when you hear your loved one's voice after a period of absence. Or your response might be knee-jerk and acted out, as when you quickly change lanes to avoid being sideswiped by some careless driver or when you first blurt out "I love you" in a new relationship.

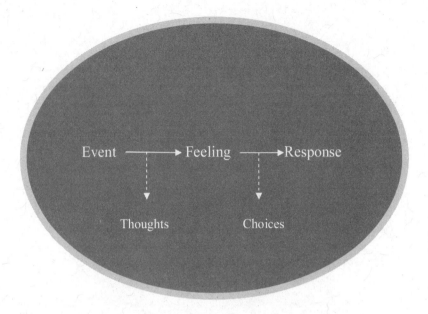

Figure 2.3: Habits of Thought

Let's take a look at some examples. Say that you're driving along the highway, minding your own business, when out of nowhere—vrooooom!—a car speeds past you, cutting in front of you unexpectedly. This is the event. You take in the information about the driving conditions and the sudden appearance and erratic behavior of the other driver and assign meaning to this behavior even before you know to be scared. In a fraction of a second your adrenaline spikes. You're scared because the event represents a danger to your life, health, and well-being. Your instinctual urge is to escape, but you're in a car, on the highway. Before you can look to see if the next lane is clear, the car that swooped down on you so abruptly has disappeared, leaving you safe but still reeling from the adrenaline rush. Your urge is blocked. Now you're angry and shaking, and you have a sudden headache.

If we examine this event broken down even more, it looks like this:

1. **Event:** A car cuts in front of you.

2. **Thought:** "Danger, Will Robinson!"

3. **Feeling:** Fear, complete with a physiological response of adrenaline with muscle tension and vascular surge (which is where the headache comes from)

4. **Urge:** To escape

Then we can break down the immediate results of this sequence by detailing another:

1. **Event:** Your urge is thwarted.

2. **Thoughts:** You expect everyone who shares the road to obey the speed limit and follow the rules; you came near to disaster or even death; you were powerless in the situation.

3. **Feeling:** Anger

4. **Urge:** To hit the steering wheel, scream, pursue the other driver, and so on

Now let's look at how this works in an example familiar to many parents. You've finally gotten to sleep when you hear the baby cry. His cries become louder and more insistent while you wait to see if he'll manage to soothe himself and go back to sleep. You think, "Oh, no, not again … I was so needing to get back to sleep," as you drag yourself out of bed and into the nursery to pick up your baby. You check his diaper, but it's dry. He continues to cry. You speak softly to him and offer breast or bottle, even though he just ate a little while ago. He refuses. You pat, rock, cuddle, and coo. Nothing works. His lip quivers. His body shakes. He's still crying.

You start to think that there is something *wrong* with this baby. You repeat the above steps. Nothing works. You start to panic. You think that your efforts *should* work—unless there is something really wrong with the baby, *your* baby. And this baby is your responsibility, so you should have prevented anything from going wrong. In fact, something may be so off-the-track wrong with him that he may die, and it will be all your fault!

You call the pediatrician's office and tell the answering service to page her right away. You keep trying to feed, burp, rock, and otherwise soothe your son. You think that there can only be two possibilities:

either there is something terribly, horribly, unthinkably wrong with this child or you are just a bad mother. Your heart is racing, and tears are running down your face. Then the phone rings, and the baby stops crying and falls asleep, all at the same time. You answer the phone, speaking softly, and answer all the standard questions the doctor puts to you. She lets you know that you can bring the baby into the office first thing in the morning, but that the situation doesn't sound like an emergency.

You hang up the phone, thinking that this job is just too hard and you're not cut out for it. After you lay the baby down, you try to go back to sleep. But now you're going back over all your efforts, trying yet again to figure out what you should have done differently. You don't realize it, but you *still* think there are only two possibilities: that there is something abnormally wrong with your baby or that you are a bad mother. In this upsetting and hopeless mental cage, you eventually fall asleep.

Exhausting, isn't it? A scene very similar to this played out recently at Sam's house. While she was calmly pacing the floor with the crying baby, her husband was yelling at her to "*do* something," the older kids were awakened by all the commotion, and the toddler joined in with the crying. Once Sam got everyone settled down, she gently kissed her husband on the forehead and suggested to him that any day now he would begin to trust that she knows what she's doing. Several days later, he apologized.

Coping Styles: Bridges to Depression

We've been examining cognitive styles and their effect on depression. Now we'll move on to what we do about our thoughts—our responses to those urges that come with emotions. So, while "cognitive styles" refers to habits of thought, how we process and think about life's dif-ficulties, "coping styles" refers to how we cope, what we do when faced with these difficulties.

Earlier I mentioned the autonomic nervous system in relation to the fight-or-flight response. In our complex, postmodern social world we still get an adrenaline rush when we feel endangered and fright-ened or powerless and angry, but we usually don't physically fight or literally run. In social relationships, we usually tackle problems ("fighting" them) or avoid them ("running"); we either level with people we care about or edit out our chagrin.

Either response can be done in a way that's helpful to you emotionally or can be handled so as to cause suffering. Especially when done thoughtfully and with compassion, addressing problems can bring new growth to your relationships. And, if you're able to resolve a conflict in your own mind and really move on, that represents growth rather than flight.

But, because we are inexperienced in either tactic and/or because our emotions around the conflict are so intense that we're afraid to move forward, we often either tackle the issue ineffectively or simply hide from it (and the emotions it comes with). Doing the latter is understood as *avoidance*. Avoidance tends to function in the context of interpersonal relations, so we'll be looking at that coping strategy in chapter 3. Here, let's examine the coping strategy that you usually do all by yourself—the repetitive, emotion-filled, and nonproductive thinking called *rumination*.

Rumination

Susan Nolen-Hoeksema is one of the scientists who noticed and was troubled by the fact that more women than men get depressed. She became curious about this and started doing research about the different ways that men and women think—especially when they are in difficult situations, situations that might constitute a risk for depression. And what she found was intriguing: men were more likely to distract when distressed, and women were more likely to persist in trying to think through interminable, unanswerable "why" questions (Nolen-Hoeksema 1987).

Other researchers have since picked up this quest and refined the understanding of what kinds of rumination lead to depression when there are other vulnerabilities present. These other vulnerabilities can be temperamental vulnerabilities, a past history of depression (remember that once a person has had an episode of major depression, the brain pathways are set to become depressed again), or the cognitive style variables we've been examining. It turns out that not just any kind of mulling things over will put you at risk—it's possible to con-template positive things and to daydream in positive ways about future events (Lavender and Watkins 2004). But when we brood over the past (which is unchangeable) or rehearse negative scenarios about a feared future, then we are ruminating (Brinker and Dozois 2009; Joormann, Dkane, and Gotlib 2006; Ciesla and Roberts 2007). And this kind of rumination gets in the way of doing the things we know are impor-tant to do to maintain healthy relationships, zaps motivation to keep working toward meaningful goals, and sucks the life out of social sup-ports (Lyubomirsky et al. 1999; Lyubomirsky and Nolen-Hoeksema 1995; Kross, Ayduk, and Mischel 2006). Rumination passes for problem solving, but it isn't. True problem solving identifies and defines a goal and articulates a clear sequence of tangible steps, of concrete actions, that you can take to solve the problem (Lyubomirsky et al. 1999). Rumination stays in your head; problem solving leads to deliberate, thoughtful action.

Rumination also interferes with sleep, and sleep deprivation turns out to be one of the most reliable predictors of depression—a factor that we will take a closer look at in chapter 5.

Changing Your Style, Changing Your Brain

If you see yourself in these descriptions and if you've started to identify some of these habits of thought in yourself, take heart. It is possible to change automatic and unconscious habits of thought—to deliber-ately rehearse new ways of interpreting events in order to release the neurotransmitters associated with positive thoughts and emotions. And if the new habit is rehearsed enough, the brain will grow a new *dendrite*—a connection between two neurons that wasn't there before (DeLange et al. 2008; Lazar et al. 2005). This means that it's not only possible to change one's brain chemistry by changing one's thoughts, it is also possible to actually change the architecture, *the connections* of the brain by changing thoughts (Hartley and Phelps 2009; DeRaedt 2006; Beauregard 2009).

In the meantime, while you are in the learning curve, medications can fill the gap and give you enough hope, enough belief that things can change, to help you be patient with yourself and keep you focused on the learning curve (Begley 2010). Medical research has documented very clearly that having negative habits of thought, living with chronic anxiety and/or depression, causes damage to specific areas of the brain (Etkin and Wager 2007; Liston, McEwen, and Casey 2008; McEwen 2009). So using medications as a stopgap, to relieve the pressure while you're learning new habits, can be a reasonable choice.

How Medications Work

Medications for depression enter through the mouth, are processed by the digestive system, pass into the bloodstream, and cross the blood–brain barrier to have a very broad, systemic effect on areas of the brain involved in troublesome emotions. *Selective serotonin reuptake inhibitors*, SSRIs, the most popular class of antidepressants in use today, are believed to work mainly by preventing the depletion (the reuptake) of one class of neurotransmitter. This preventative function presumably makes the positive neurotransmitters more abundant and more available.

Medications can be very helpful in treating depression because they often work relatively quickly. But, perhaps more importantly, medications have been shown to lessen the damaging impact of stress hormones, the neurochemicals that accompany negative thinking, on the brain (D'Sa and Duman 2002; Radley et al. 2004; Shansky et al. 2009). Because medications can take effect more quickly and learning to change automatic and unconscious habits of thought can take some time, clients who are suicidal, who are experiencing severe and prolonged sleep disturbance, or who are losing touch with reality and at risk for psychosis may need to be hospitalized or medicated before psychotherapy can be most useful.

Intentionally changing one's habits of thought is more difficult than taking a pill, but the effect of this hard work is more specific to thoughts, feelings, and behavior, while medications necessarily affect body and brain and always have some side effects. Research using fMRI technology has repeatedly shown that, over time, changes in habits of thought and changes in behavior learned in cognitive behavioral therapy show up as visible changes in the brain: "The data, for example in depression, panic disorder, phobia and obsessive compulsive disorder (OCD), clearly suggested that a change in patients' symptoms and maladaptive behavior at the mind level with psychological techniques is accompanied with functional brain changes in relevant brain circuits. In many studies, cognitive therapies and drug therapies achieved therapeutic gains through the same neural pathways although the two forms of treatment may still have different mechanisms of action" (Kumari 2006, 61).

Outcome research, research comparing the effectiveness of cognitive behavioral psychotherapy versus medications, has consistently shown that both are effective initially and that psychotherapy is *at least* as effective as medication, but the combination of cognitive behavioral psychotherapy together with medications is more effective than either treatment alone (Boren, Leventhal, and Pigott 2009; DeRubeis et al. 1999; DeRubeis et al. 2005).

Of course, it's always preferable to prevent depression from happening a first time than to keep it from progressing or from recurring, and if you're already depressed, isn't it good to think that once you learn these skills you can use them to prevent a future occurrence? In studies comparing relapse rates for patients who stopped taking medications versus those who finished cognitive behavioral therapy for depression, the patients on medication relapsed within a year after the treatment was withdrawn. Those who "graduated" from therapy kept what they learned and stayed well, especially if the CBT included a behavior-activation component (Hollon et al. 2005; Dobson et al. 2008; Dimidjian et al. 2006). *Behavioral activation*, of course, refers to something that gets you moving—which is why it's so important to do homework and actually try out new behaviors. This is one reason I've included assignments at the end of each chapter.

Exercises for Chapter 2

The first step to stopping automatic habits of thought is to recognize what they are. When we first learn something new, we go through a predictable series of stages. First we don't know what we don't know. Then we begin to realize just how much there is to learn—we become aware of what we don't know. Then, as we learn, we go through a stage where we know more than we think we do. Finally, we arrive at proficiency, the stage where we know and we know that we know. Whatever your habits of thought are, you've rehearsed them so many times that they are now automatic and they feel true. Therefore, they go unquestioned. And typically you will notice your feelings before you become aware of the thoughts, even though the thoughts really came first.

If you can interrupt the progression between event, thought, and feeling, you will gain more control over your feelings. But, if this is a new skill for you, you'll probably need a little bit of help in learning how to break the progression down to its elements. We'll go ahead and work on that now.

Exercise 1: Identifying Habits of Thought

Grab your notebook, turn it sideways, and draw three columns. Use the Event, Story, Feelings Worksheet as a model. Make the middle column bigger than the two side columns. Label the top of the first column "Event." Label the middle column "Story Line (Interpretation)." Label the third column "Feelings."

For this exercise, we'll be working backward with a memory of a feeling. But, once you get the hang of it, you'll be able to pause at the moment when you're having some strong emotion, pull out your notebook, and follow this example. Catching yourself between event and thoughts, or between thoughts and feelings, can save you many painful emotions.

As a first step, think back to a time you had a very strong emotion. It might be helpful to try to recall a fairly recent event (so the thought progression is clearer), but using a very strong emotion from any time may work out just fine. Remembering this strong feeling, write about how it felt in as much detail as you can muster. (Write these details in the third column on your homemade worksheet, under "Feelings.") Start with the feeling's name, then what that emotion's signature is in *your* body.

Once you've named and described the feeling, hop over to the first column and jot down whatever you remember about what was going on at the time this emotion welled up in you. It doesn't matter whether you think the events surrounding your emotion are relevant to your feelings—sometimes they are and sometimes they're not. Just practice describing what was leading up to your emotion as objectively as you can.

Once you've filled in these two columns, now (and only now) it's time to work on the middle column. Pause and reflect on what went through your mind between the event and the feeling. This is the part where you just write down your stream of consciousness without editing and without judging whether you think the thoughts were true, relevant, important, or meaningful.

Once you've filled in this column, step back and take a look at your statements objectively. I know it may sound strange, but there is actually a sizeable body of literature about how helpful a writing exercise can be in learning to regulate emotions, and I have found this particular structure to be very helpful.

Figure 2.4: Event, Story, Feelings Worksheet

Event	Story Line (Interpretation)	Feelings
Put honey on pacifier Found out honey can cause botulism in babies.	I almost killed my baby. I'm a terrible mother. I'm so dumb. My baby deserves better.	Scared, angry, sad, worthless, disappointed, hopeless, discouraged Heart beats fast, palms sweaty Chest is tight; feel like crying

Exercise 2: Connecting Feelings to Thoughts

Now take a closer look at your worksheet. Going back over your stories (interpretations), check for common cognitive distortions that may be contributing to your negative feelings about each event. You might even try having someone else look over your stories since they likely seem so reasonable and true to you. Use a highlighter to identify common unhelpful habits of thought. Consider which might be:

- Global thinking or overly inclusive, blanket statements

- Binary thinking, meaning either/or, black/white, all/none statements

- Assumptions of causality when you really don't know

- Implied standards of perfection

- External locus of control

- Internalized statements of blame

Exercise 3: Trying On New Ways of Thinking

Next, practice rewriting your stories in your notebook. There, you'll be sure to have enough room to be detailed. Here are some tips for the rewrite:

- Identify what you really don't know and admit it.

- Admit when you're not to blame because you only had partial control.

- Try to guesstimate just how much influence you had in the situation using percentages (98 percent control? 50 percent?).

- Admit when you might have had influence (but not control) that you overlooked.

- Now consider this: you're only 50 percent of any given interaction with another human being.

How do your emotions change when you rewrite the explanations? If the change is the same for each of the stories, you can generalize. Or, be detailed for each story, considering how your emotions change in each situation.

Exercise 4:
Get to Know Your Emotions

Information is power, and the more information you have about your own emotional experiences (particularly the connection between your thoughts and your feelings), the more power you will have to modify your emotional experience when you need to.

So with your notebook turned sideways, draw three columns (using the Getting to Know Your Emotions Worksheet as a guide). This time label one column "Emotion Name," the other column "Body Signature," and the last one "Soothing Strategies." We'll be working on the first column here and the other two in a bit.

Right now, list some emotions you've had recently. For each of the emotions you can think of (I've provided a list to get you started), think of a time when you felt that emotion. Make your memory as vivid and detailed as possible.

Figure 2.5: Getting to Know Your Emotions Worksheet

Emotion Name	Body Signature	Soothing Strategies
Annoyed	Tension in back of neck Tight jaw Tight shoulders	Stretching exercises Breathing exercises Focusing on letting go

Example Emotions

Basic:

Anger

Sorrow

Fear

Love

Joy

Nuanced:

> Annoyed
>
> Wistful
>
> Worried
>
> Sympathy
>
> Amused
>
> Determined
>
> Put out
>
> Sorry for
>
> Impatient
>
> Compassion
>
> Touched
>
> Tickled

Feel free to add to this list. The more nuanced you get, the better.

Exercise 5: Develop Categories and Criteria

Referring back to the exercises you've just worked on, are there particular emotions that seem indistinguishable to you? If so, which ones?

1. Write them down in your notebook.

2. Describe how they are alike—be as detailed and specific as you can.

3. Now look for subtle clues as to how they are different. (Hint: pay attention to the stories.)

The more you know the specific signatures of your emotions, the more power you will have to step back, validate yourself, and choose your response more carefully.

Exercise 6: Develop Awareness of Body Tension

Now let's work with the second column of figure 2.5, "Body Signature." Try to identify exactly where in your body you feel each emotion. The more familiar you become with your body's code for signaling emotions, the more quickly you will be able to move from deciphering the emotion to solving problems and the clearer your decisions will be.

Come up with several ways to soothe body tension that work for you:

- Breathing deeply

- Cultivating mindfulness of the body

- Listening to a hypnosis or relaxation tape/CD

- Counting to ten

- Humming a familiar tune

- Singing out loud

- Taking a hot shower or bath

- Exercising really hard

- Watching a funny movie

- Thinking funny or particularly loving thoughts

Come up with several "mantras" or story lines to help you refocus on the present. For instance, you might try "All I can do is do all I can," or "I'm only one half of any interaction."

Exercise 7: Distinguishing Degrees of Excellence

We all have limited resources—time, emotional reserves, and funds. Consequently, we all have to learn to make choices that take real limits into account. If we don't take a hard look at the limits of our resources we can easily fall into the trap of imagining that we can be excellent at everything. And that is a formula for failure.

This exercise is designed to help you set realistic expectations about what you can reasonably expect to accomplish. Go ahead and start by identifying three things that it's okay for you to fail at. Try to be specific about things that you may have trouble with or have been hard on yourself about in the past.

1.

2.

3.

Identify three things that you can allow yourself to be "good enough" at:

1.

2.

3.

When is it okay to settle for good enough? How did you choose the items above? How do you decide when to settle for good enough? Be specific.

Identify three things that you had to learn but that you now do well. Now think back to the time before you knew how to do each thing and remember how you went about learning it. How did you start? How did your learning progress? Try to identify the stages of your learning curve for each.

1.

2.

3.

How do you know when you do well? Be specific. If you have trouble with this, ask others how they know they are doing well and what criteria they use. But remember, you're not obligated to adopt the criteria of others.

Exercise 8: Count the Cost of Various Choices

Identify something you wish to do better as a parent (a learning goal). How much will it cost you to improve? Estimate time, money, and emotional energy in your cost analysis. For example, I would love to be an excellent gardener. But the truth of the matter is that I don't have enough interest in learning about different plants or enough passion about the actual process of gardening to put up with the learning curve involved in digging, planting, and tending things in my garden. So I outsourced the landscaping (when I reached that item on my priority list), and I do only the bare essentials. If I were to take on the task of learning to become an excellent gardener (I know that I would aspire to be really good, not just okay), it would cost me time, money, and emotional energy. When I look at the prospect realistically, I can see that those resources just aren't available right now, so I decide to let this be a possible goal for the future.

What aspirations do you have as a parent that you actually have the wherewithal to achieve? Write the answer down here and/or in your notebook.

Exercise 9: Create an Improvement Plan

Using the learning goal you chose in exercise 8, it's time to create an improvement plan. First, list your goal one more time. Learning to fence was one of my goals.

I want to learn how to fence.

Next, break down this goal into three to five big steps you'll have to take to achieve it.

1. Get as much information as possible on local resources.

2. Contact possible places where fencing is taught to adults.

3. Go to the first class.

4. Watch to see if I really like it.

5. Sign up for a class and pay fees.

Now, take a close look at each of these large steps and break each one down into many small steps. Make these steps as small as you like—remember, each step you can cross off, you can credit yourself for a success. So, don't make the steps so small that you will feel ridiculous crossing them off, but make sure they're small enough to do fairly easily. (You may want to get some help breaking down your bigger steps. Sometimes a loved one can see how to proceed with small steps more clearly, as they're not as affected by the pressure of the goal.) Write your small steps in your notebook, so you'll have plenty of space.

Note: If you decide this is just too much work right now, perhaps it means the benefits do not outweigh the costs and you would do better to go easy on yourself. You can create a learning plan when it feels more comfortable for you. Remember, you have limited emotional resources right now.

CHAPTER 3

The Social Side of Depression

Without friends no one would choose to live, though he had all other goods.

Aristotle

So far in our work, we've looked at biological aspects of the thoughts and feelings that go to make up what we call "postpartum depression" and we've seen how certain habits of thought can cause depression. Now we'll look at the social side of life—how relationships influence thoughts and feelings contributing to happiness or not. Relationships, at various levels from nuclear family to community and social support, are vitally important to mental health. And, as it turns out, how you relate to others plays a major role in your level of happiness and satisfaction—as a new parent and as a human being.

The Importance of Belonging

The need to belong is primal. The human infant is dependent on others, adults of the species, for a very long time, and throughout history individual humans have also been dependent on groups of other humans for survival. This need for acceptance by other human beings is hardwired into our brains, encoded into the most basic apparatus of our survival. While many psychological theorists emphasize the importance of the mother–infant bond (often called attachment) in the development of personality and psychopathology (Ainsworth 1969, 11–12; Ainsworth and Bell 1970; Bell and Ainsworth 1972), others emphasize the life-long need to belong to a larger clan, underscoring the importance of group membership well beyond infancy (Murphy 1949; Sullivan 1955; Baumeister and Leary 1995). Both are certainly important in different ways, and the two are intertwined in ways that are, frankly, separable: "Studying the interrelations of temperament and of cultural coercions, we reach a point where practically the entire cultural picture must be studied to say anything meaningful about a person" (Murphy 1949, 16). The need for social inclusion is so extensive and so powerful that the threat of social rejection and resulting loneliness can actually measurably decrease intelligence (Baumeister, Twenge, and Nuss 2002). And group exclusion impairs self-regulation, leading to decreased pro-social behavior and increased aggression (Baumeister et al. 2005; Twenge et al. 2001; Twenge et al. 2007).

Human beings are born into families that are embedded in communities which, in turn, are ensconced in a culture. These groups vary in how widespread and how interconnected they are. Because belonging to a social group is such a powerful need, human culture devises rules, called *mores* (pronounced moh'rays), which amount to agreed-upon codes of conduct meant to ease communal living. These rules, understood and accepted by those in the group, help make living in close association with other human beings a positive experience, keeping friction to a minimum (LeVine and New 2008; Stix 1996). As cultures become very large, some of those mores get codified into laws and are enforced with greater force than mere disapproval.

As you might expect, cultural groups and their norms do change over time. For instance, once a group becomes larger than about 150 people, problems tend to erupt, and a group will often subdivide (Gladwell 2000). Since people tend to confuse *consensual truth*, which is what is agreed upon by a group (examples include values like human equality or that democracy is the best form of government) with *absolute truth* (examples include gravity—a group doesn't have to believe in the force of gravity for it to be true), when different groups with different codes for conducting social relationships come into contact with one another, tensions tend to arise. Throughout history, wars have sometimes resulted from this tension. But after a war is over, the groups that fought tend to mingle and intermarry so that the codes for conducting social life change again (Gladwell 2000).

Despite an increasingly global economy and worldwide blending of cultures by media, the need to belong is hardwired (Baumeister and Leary 1995). Jean Twenge, a psychologist who has spent her academic career studying the changes in personality profiles of Americans over several decades, notes that Americans are more isolated and lonely now than in previous generations—at least the generations for which we have data (her data goes back, in some cases, to the 1920s and 1930s) (Twenge et al. 2008; Twenge 2001; Twenge and Campbell 2009). Dr. Twenge's books *Generation Me* and *The Narcissism Epidemic* document these social changes in great detail, which I will not attempt to duplicate here (Twenge 2006; Twenge and Campbell 2009). Suffice it to say that as a culture, we have grown increasingly focused on the individual and increasingly disconnected from others. And this state of affairs has a significant impact on parenting. According to Twenge, this generation of new parents is "malnourished from eating a junk-food diet of instant messages, e-mail, and phone calls rather than the healthy food of live, in-person interaction" and is four times lonelier than their parents' generation was at this age (2006, 110). As you might imagine, these feelings of loneliness and isolation can have a marked impact on your experience of parenthood and your overall feeling of well-being.

Rites of Passage

Pervasive isolation means that many of us move through our lives without the touch points our ancestors relied upon. For instance, as we reach transitional points in our lives, we have only diluted markers to honor these experiences and support us as we move into a new phase of life. We've lost many of our rites of passage, and as new parents, we may feel at sea in the seemingly unacknowledged magnitude of the change we're undergoing.

In traditional societies where the importance of belonging was recognized, social rituals existed to help members make life transitions (Erikson 1950). The transition from childhood to adulthood, for example, was marked and celebrated by rituals of passage for coming of age; the transition from single adult to family unit marked by socially meaningful marriage rituals. And the transition to parenthood was also typically marked by ritual and prescribed forms of social support (Bibring 1959). But in our modern society, all we have left is the wedding industry; we lack truly meaningful rituals for coming of age and for the transition to parenthood. So, teenagers invent their own ways of establishing group status and create their own rites of passage; new parents get a baby shower and maybe a covered dish. But the deeply meaningful social function of rite and ritual are lost, and what remains is woefully inadequate. The rituals of traditional societies not only helped to celebrate life transitions and give social meaning to these normative events, they also served to impart security by limiting ambiguity and by imparting status. The new spouse's or new parent's social status, meaning the sense of being important and valuable to the group as a whole, depended on assuming the adult roles of parents and responsibilities of family (Bibring 1959; Erikson 1950; Cowan and Cowan 1995). But in our individualistic society, we expect to go it alone; we are not supposed to care what other people think. The result is isolation, a loss of meaning, and profound depression. And depression is affecting this generation of parents more than any previous generation. "Only 1 percent to 2 percent of Americans born before 1915 experienced a major depressive episode during their lifetime, even though they lived through the Great Depression and two world wars. Today the lifetime rate of major depression is ten times higher—between 15 percent and 20 percent" (Twenge 2006, 105).

Family and Society in Historical Context

These days, the norm is the nuclear family—mother, father, and child or children living in the same house, while extended family members live elsewhere. This setup is seen as representative of economic success. In other words, we have enough resources to enable each family unit to have its own living space. However, what we gain in comporting to this norm may be relatively paltry when compared to the resulting loss of social support and increased depression.

In her book *The Way We Never Were*, sociologist Stephanie Coontz methodically demonstrates that the nuclear family is a modern construction, and the nostalgia often expressed in the popular press for some past time when marriages were allegedly stable and children supposedly grew up with two parents is misplaced. Those golden days are a myth that is simply not supported by historical or sociological evidence (1992). Colonial families were highly unstable simply because mortality rates were so high that the average marriage lasted less than twelve years (Coontz 1992). Any child lucky enough to survive to age twenty-one had a 30 to 50 percent chance of having lost at least one parent (and that statistic was higher in the South). Victorians of the 1830s and 1840s didn't fare much better—especially so for the less than middle class. Slave families were regularly split up and sold separately. Children were put to work in sweatshops with little or no opportunity for education, much less affection and family cohesion. Let us remember that "[f]or every nineteenth-century middle-class family that protected its wife and child within the family circle, there was an Irish or German girl scrubbing floors in that middle-class home, a Welsh boy mining coal to keep the home-baked goodies warm, a black girl doing the family laundry, a black mother and child picking cotton to be made into clothes for the family, and a Jewish or an Italian daughter in a sweatshop making 'ladies' dresses or artificial flowers for the family to purchase" (Coontz 1992, 11–12). This sentimentality about times past is often linked to our modern divorce rates, but what is overlooked is that "the 50 percent divorce rate estimates are calculated in terms of a forty-year period and ... many marriages in the past were terminated well before that date by the death of one partner" (Coontz 1992, 16). Historically, mother–infant bonding was often a luxury, but belonging to a group was essential for survival. Even today I frequently meet immigrants who have left young children behind to be cared for by family and community, adults who have been raised by many relatives, and various others for whom the essential elements of family are, or have been, met through a sense of belonging to a group.

Essential Ingredients of Belonging

Belonging is a fundamental need, and it is not fulfilled by any random kind of belonging. People have a powerful need to belong to social groups that involve *lasting, positive, significant,* and *reciprocal* relationships with other people (Baumeister and Leary 1995). In order to satisfy this need, people must have emotionally pleasant interactions with several other people. These relationships must be meaningful, in that they involve genuine caring; they must be stable, involving the same people over time; the caring must be reciprocal, not just a one-way kind of relationship like those involving professionals or hired caregivers; and the relationship must involve frequent live contact over time, and it must involve some form of human touch (Hertenstein et al. 2009). Without this kind of group belonging, people become sick and exhibit severe pathology that places them at a great disadvantage in terms of survival (Baumeister and Leary 1995). Without this kind of belonging, very specific areas of the brain atrophy (Gianaros et al. 2007).

The need to belong to a group is fundamental and produces a primal drive in people. But the ability for people to find and maintain lasting social connections that meet this need is not adequately facilitated by the nuclear family or the modern emphasis on individuality, and it is severely challenged by the structure of our professional lives (Twenge, Catanese, and Baumeister 2003; Baumeister and Leary 1995; Twenge 2006). Social expectations and work obligations no longer support the kind of community that this need presupposes.

New parents are often caught in the crosshairs between the fundamental need for belonging and the realities of modern life. All too often, they are left bereft of the protections once afforded by belonging to community. These benefits, so very crucial in times of stress, include:

- Knowing that you don't have to go it alone

- Understanding that you can (and are expected to) call on help in times of need

- Playing enough different roles within the group to feel valued without feeling overwhelmed

◆ Having the sense of security that results from knowing what the social expectations are and how to fulfill these expectations successfully

Contrary to many modern notions, science has shown over and over again that human beings are hardwired for community, and being lonely or alone is a risk factor for anxiety, depression, and a host of physical ills.

Belonging and Depression

As I've mentioned, without a strong sense of belonging, without help (or the possibility of help) from a wider community, a new parent is at significant risk of feelings of isolation and of being overwhelmed. And a next logical jump is to descend to feelings of sadness and even toward depression. Thus, the way we structure our social context—not only on a personal level but at the level of our society and culture— can have a significant effect on whether new parents are at risk for depression (Twenge, Campbell, and Foster 2003; Longsdon, McBride, and Birkhimer 1994; Stemp, Turner, and Noh 1986).

If social and cultural variables are important risk factors for developing depression in general and postpartum depression in particular, then we would expect to find differences in the rates of depression and in postpartum depression in different cultures. And, in fact, we do. Not only are rates of depression different across different cultures (Simon et al. 2002; Simon et al. 2004), not only are there some cultures where postpartum depression is virtually unknown (Harkness 1987), but perhaps most interestingly, depression increases as a culture becomes increasingly Westernized (Yapko 2009; Marsella et al. 1985; Kleinman and Good 1985). And in this country, Hispanics have remarkably low (2.4 percent) rates of postpartum depression (Wei et al. 2008). Can it be a mere coincidence that the Hispanic subculture in the United States also values and emphasizes extensive family and social ties or that Hispanics often live in multigenerational households? Something about our Western industrialized social structures in general and American culture in particular seems to promote postpartum depression in men and women.

The Happiness Literature

Epidemiologists study how diseases spread. Sociologists study social trends and patterns of social influence. Recently, James Fowler and Nicholas Christakis, two social scientists from U.C. Berkeley and Harvard, respectively, borrowed the data analysis methods common in epidemiology to study the patterns of social relationships in a group. Instead of medical information—things like blood pressure, cholesterol levels, and heart attacks—they were looking for health behaviors— things like happiness, smoking, and obesity (Christakis and Fowler 2007; Christakis and Fowler 2008; Fowler and Christakis 2008). Their results are fascinating. They found that healthy behaviors like quitting smoking, staying trim and fit, and being happy are just as contagious as viruses. Christakis and Fowler were able to show that people influenced one another's health in powerful ways through close, regular contact over many years. And the opposite was also true. Those who isolated themselves through their negativity and unhealthy behaviors clustered together in small cells and became marginalized from the larger group—with predictable declines to their emotional and physical health. In order to maintain optimal health, people need to belong to stable groups and to have genuine caring relationships that involve frequent, meaningful and emotionally pleasant interactions with several people, the same several people, over a long time. Meanwhile, new parents are more isolated than ever before, straining the relationship and putting them at risk for postpartum depression (Twenge, Campbell, and Foster 2003; Gianino 2008). The mechanisms behind just how people influence one another emotionally remain somewhat obscure, but research from several different fields offers important clues.

Emotion Contagion

Neuroscientists recently made a breakthrough discovery when they found that the brain contains highly specialized neurons called *mirror neurons* that fire both when the subject (a person or other animal) observes another person or animal engaging in a behavior, and when they engage in it themselves. For example, if you observe someone smiling, there is a part of your brain that activates, and some of the neurons in this part of your brain are the exact same ones that activate when you smile. So, of course, seeing someone smile (or frown) *feels* a lot like you're the one doing the smiling (or frowning) too. In other words, "observing the actions and tactile sensations of others activates premotor, posterior parietal and somatosensory regions in the brain of the observer, which are also active when performing similar movements and feeling similar sensations" (Bastiaansen, Thioux, and Keysers 2009, 2391). This is one of two processes that researchers believe is the basis for empathy. It is also one basis for emotional contagion. *Emotional contagion* refers to our tendency to pick up and become "infected" by the emotions of others. Thus, depression is contagious in ways that are analogous to how viruses are spread, although the mechanism is different (Yapko 1999; Yapko 2009). Examples of the contagion of depression span a wide range. For example, college students who get a depressed roommate are significantly more likely to end up depressed and with poor study habits than college students who find themselves rooming with a happy person (Joiner 1994). When one spouse becomes depressed it is also very difficult for the other spouse to remain happy (Meignan et al. 1999; Benazon 2000; Benazon and Coyne 2000). For one thing, depressed people tend to find happy people irritating. So, they try to elicit sympathy in ways that, instead, kills the joy of those they come in contact with. (We'll be examining these unhelpful strategies more closely later in the chapter.)

Knowing that depression is contagious, you can learn to be on guard to avoid spreading your low mood to others and to be less vulnerable to getting caught up in another's depression. And, as we've seen, helping the people around you from sinking will buoy you up at the same time. What you communicate and how you communicate are two things that are definitely under your control—even when you are depressed. Learning to take control of this important area can give you a powerful means of protecting yourself from deepening a bad day into a full-blown depression and can help you prevent relapse and contagion.

Loneliness and Social-Network Changes

Whereas in other cultures and in times past in our own culture, the transition to parenthood marked a passage into *increased* social connection and social status, today's parents find themselves more isolated than ever. Friends they thought they would have forever drop out, and networks become smaller and more homogenous—consisting mainly of close family members and the parents of other small children (Bost et al. 2002). In order to better understand the social supports of married people with children as compared to the social supports of child-free married couples, researchers examined data from 2,194 couples who responded to the 1978 American Quality of Life Survey. Previous research had found that childless couples were the more socially isolated, but in this study "[t]here was a higher level of marital support among childless people than among parents of younger children" (Ishii-Kuntz and Seccombe 1989, 777). Given social trends since 1978, we can only assume this isolation is even deeper now than thirty years ago.

As the social network constricts, what is left mostly consists of female relatives and a few other mothers with most of the pressure for support landing squarely on the marriage itself. This can be an uncomfortable change or a welcome surprise, depending largely on what kind of relationship these parents have with female relatives. "Interactions with spouse and with kin are based on intimacy as well as formal obligations for goods and services. Support from spouse and kin is therefore likely to reflect intimacy and a long-term relationship. Interaction with friends, on the other hand, is based on reciprocity. Bonds of friendship, as a rule, develop between people who view each other as equals and who have common interests and experiences that are freely shared" (Ishii-Kuntz and Seccombe 1989, 778). Thus, couples find that they are more likely to socialize with a few other couples who also have small children and with family members who are more likely to be supportive and involved with them (Bost et al. 2002). Women are more likely to turn to their mothers and to female relatives—aunts, grandmothers, sisters—during the transition to parenthood, while men often wish they could turn to their fathers for advice about

fathering but are more likely to want to "offer their own child a different fathering experience" than they had (Deave, Johnson, and Ingram
2008, 4). The tendency toward social isolation of couples when children are small can be particularly difficult for lesbian mothers, who
might already have strained relationships with family because of their
sexual orientation and choice to have children in an unconventional
arrangement (Goldberg and Sayer 2006). It is also particularly difficult
for people who live far from or no longer have close kin. Gay men also
find their social networks changing when they become parents. They
find themselves more alienated from the gay community and are more
likely to begin affiliating with heterosexual couples with children of
similar ages to their own (Gianino 2008). All this suggests that modern
parents must be very intentional about cultivating their social connections, and, in order to be most successful at managing this shift, you
will need to mind your social skills and pay close attention to habits
of relating.

Habits of Relating

Earlier, I mentioned that the way we relate to other people can affect
our mental and physical well-being. It makes sense: if other people can
influence our moods and our physical health, how we interact with
these people would play an important part in the equation. We've also
seen how some cultures seek to regularize some of our social interactions to make sure expectations are managed and behavior is predictable and helpful. Rituals and rites of passage serve these functions, and
their relative disappearance in our modern culture means that we are
much more on our own in terms of how we relate to others and how
we rally support. The pre-birth baby showers and post-delivery covered
dishes dropped off at the house might not be enough social support for
some new parents. Having the self-awareness to know your own needs
for support and the social skills to elicit the support you need can be
tricky (Ravitz 2003). As with most human activities, habits of relating can be complex. But understanding how you operate with other
people—and whether the strategies you use to get your needs met are
effective—is the first step toward getting the help you need.

The Avoidant Coping Style and Social Isolation

In chapter 2 we examined different coping styles that tended to create a vulnerability to depression. As you'll recall, these were a ruminative style and an avoidant style. While the ruminative coping style has more to do with your habits of thought, the avoidant coping style affects your habits of relating—whether you reach out for social support, and how.

Ambivalence can be defined as the uncomfortable process of oscillating between approach and avoidance. Rumination happens when the approach-oriented coping fails to accomplish the goal of solving a problem and instead leaves the person going over and over the same mental ground, rehearsing worst-case scenarios without ever coming to a conclusion that leads to action. Avoidance is the other side of this dilemma. Avoidant coping can involve cognitive strategies like not thinking about (and therefore not solving) problems or giving in to the urge to withdraw from social contact. Let's take a look at how this plays out with one couple.

After Terri's paternity leave was over and he returned to work, Morgan found herself at home alone with the baby, bored to tears. She was tired because the baby still wasn't sleeping through the night, so she stayed in her PJs and napped whenever the baby did. When Terri got home at night the dishes were piled up in the sink, the bed was unmade, and Morgan was still wearing the same thing she had on when he left in the morning. None of their friends had kids yet, and all of her girlfriends worked. Several had new relationships that kept them busy, so after the excitement of the birth was over, they disappeared into their own lives. Morgan knew it was time to become a "mother," but she had no idea where to start; the task of re-creating herself was overwhelming, and so she did nothing. She avoided the whole issue.

Avoidance leads to social isolation, resentment, and blame-centered communications that breed more social isolation and depression. When Terri asked what Morgan did all day, she got defensive and accused him of having it easy because he got to go to work. Rumination is one way to maintain depression; avoidance is another; lashing out and blaming instead of asking for the help you need is yet another. Depressed people tend to do all of these things, and making small but consistent changes in each of these areas can significantly improve depression by reducing social isolation and improving the quality of social relationships. It is important to know your own needs for care and to communicate those needs in ways that don't drive loved ones and potential caregivers away (Ravitz 2003; Crowe and Luty 2005).

Morgan was so blinded by her depression she didn't even know that what she needed was more social contact. Once she identified that she needed to be around people, that she needed friends, she was able to start constructing a plan. She began by developing a routine for herself—get up, get showered and dressed, and leave the house with the baby. She made a list of places she could go that were nearby: the grocery store, the local coffee shop, and the mall. She went with explicit instructions to strike up conversations with strangers and to make eye contact and smile at anyone who initiated a conversation with her. She decided to talk to the baby about the things that she saw. Not only did it entertain her child, but chattering in a pleasant tone of voice about things outside of herself helped her notice more of her surroundings. Talking in this way also developed her sense of connection with the baby, even though he couldn't carry his end of the conversation yet.

During one of her excursions Morgan passed a church and saw that it was hosting a MOPs ("mothers of preschoolers") program. Curious, she decided to check it out and made a point to attend the next meeting. It took some doing—she was nervous about going out with her young son and a little shy about meeting other moms. But she made herself go, and soon began to meet women who also had infants at home. This was a first step in helping her social world grow. And social isolation can afflict men too after baby.

Collins also found himself isolated after his baby, Kayden, was born. Before he and Bing married, he was a freelance videographer and she was a high-paid accountant at a large corporate accounting firm. When Bing's maternity leave was up, Collins decided to stay at home with Kayden. Collins' work flow was unpredictable, and he often earned less than day care would cost in their city, so it made practical sense that he take charge of caring for the baby in these early days.

One big difference between Collins and Morgan, our two stay-at-home parents, is that Collins gets "points" in the social world for being the full-time dad. Everywhere he goes with Kayden he gets kudos for being the nurturing man, and people flock to him to ask him about his experience as a full-time daddy. Being the entrepreneurial type, Collins started the stay-at-home-dads support group in his area. Morgan lost all her specialness once the belly was gone and felt reduced to "just" a stay-at-home mom. Collins was getting a lot of social support by virtue of cultural expectations about gender. Morgan, on the other hand, had resources available to her, but she had to overcome her avoidance tendencies in order to find them.

The Depression–Rejection Link

Since belonging is such a powerful human need, naturally, the fear of rejection is also a powerful driving force. It makes sense that the loss of identity and social support that comes with early parenthood would undermine many parents' feelings of security and belonging. Therefore, new parents, especially those prone to depression for all the reasons we've examined, may be even more sensitive to rejection than they were before parenthood.

How a person manages his or her fears of rejection turns out to be an important variable in depression, marital satisfaction, *and* happiness. People who "anxiously anticipate, readily perceive, and over-react to rejection" actually increase the probability of experiencing rejection—they paradoxically cause the very thing they fear the most (Ayduk, Downey, and Kim 2001, 868). There are three habits of relating that reliably lead to depression. These three habits of relating are excessive reassurance seeking, negative self-verification, and hostile reactivity, and each one contributes to creating the very rejection that a depressed person most fears and the social isolation that then maintains depression.

One way to create a self-fulfilling prophecy of rejection is through *excessive reassurance seeking*, also known as ERS (Ayduk et al. 2000; Starr and Davila 2008). Excessive reassurance seeking repels others instead of drawing them closer. Deliberately prompting others for negative feedback typically confirms negative self-perceptions and is therefore called *negative self verification* (Giesler, Josephs, and Swann 1996; Pettit and Joiner 2006b). Finally, people who are rejection sensitive also often react to others defensively, creating the rejection they fear by projecting hostility. This habit of relating is called *hostile reactivity* and reliably produces the social isolation that leads to or maintains depression (Ayduk, Mischel, and Downey 2002; King-Casas et al. 2008).

Asking For What You Need but Missing the Mark

While mirror neurons are one of the biological reasons for the contagiousness of emotions, social factors—like how we relate to others—can also communicate emotions and play a part in attracting or repelling the social contact we need. Excessive reassurance seeking is one of those. Lost in the fog of depression, it can be hard to believe anything good about yourself. But this creates a painful dilemma for those you love. Depressed people need a lot of reassurance. The problem is, they often don't believe the reassurance they get. It's as if rejecting positive information about yourself is pleasurable in some perverse way. And it is, in the sense that validation feels good and being right feels comforting. Meanwhile, those who love the depressed person eventually become exasperated by the repeated demands for reassurance, frustrated that their reassurances do not seem to provide any relief and tired of falling into the same trap. For example:

Depressed person:	I'm a terrible person. I know you can't possibly love me...not really.
Lover of depressed person:	You're not a terrible person, and I do love you...
Depressed person:	You're just saying that.
Lover of depressed person:	Okay, fine. Suit yourself.

In this dialogue, the depressed person has just allowed his or her own self-doubt, a product of depression, to create a self-fulfilling prophecy of rejection. Overlooking the fundamental fact that he or she is not the only person in the relationship or the only one with feelings, the depressed person has just left the other person feeling pained and powerless. If you're this depressed person, then you have just traded the opportunity for relief for the comfort of predictability; the illusion of control.

Research shows that there is a certain relief that comes with validation, even when what is being validated is negative information about yourself (Kraus and Chen 2009; Chen, English, and Peng 2006).

But along with the satisfaction of validation comes a very unpleasant feeling. Because the satisfaction of validation and the unpleasantness of the negative information occur together, a cycle is set in motion that keeps repeating itself (Burns et al. 2006; Haeffel, Voelz, and Joiner 2007). It's a little bit like the cravings of an addict: the "drug" is confirmation, but it's negative so it's harmful too. This catch-22 is a little piece of hell on earth—for depressed people *and* for those who love them (Pettit and Joiner 2006a, 2006b). It seems that asking for reassurance is a normal and natural aspect of all kinds of relationships (Weary, Jordan, and Hill 1985). But when the depressed reassurance-seeker *disbelieves* the feedback, as depressed people tend to do, then the person she is seeking reassurance from is likely to interpret the repetition as evidence that the depressed person doesn't believe him or value his opinion (Swann and Bosson 1999). And therein lies the rub—as well as the contagion.

If you are depressed and you keep asking for reassurance, you are quite unintentionally doing something potentially damaging to your relationships and frustrating to the people you love and who love you. You're telling these loved ones that you don't believe them. What happens when you contradict someone over and over? What happens when you keep telling someone that you don't believe them? They get frustrated. They feel powerless. They may eventually get depressed too. They don't want to be around you because, deep inside, they think, "Oh, no—here we go again." You are contradicting the basic self-concept of the people you love, people who think of themselves as honest, sincere, loving, and believable. They want to be helpful but keep finding that, no matter what they say or how many times they say it, you are going to dismiss them.

To circumvent this sad dynamic, consider this rule of thumb: When you're unsure of how you're coming across in a social situation and you need a reality check, a little reassurance that your compass is working, you get to ask for reassurance *once*. Then, instead of going back to the well, replay the conversation in your mind. Make a point to remind yourself that looking for evidence of imperfection in yourself is a function of depression, and that it's bound to be a self-fulfilling prophecy. You see only what you're looking for—that you're no good. What you really need is the opposite: information about what you're doing right or well. Finally, you get to make up your mind to pay attention instead to the exceptions—the evidence that challenges your negative beliefs. Any one of us can find plenty of evidence of flaws in ourself; appreciation is what's hard to come by. But blanket praise, praise that is undeserved, never did anyone any good. So, instead you have to be very, very specific in what you pay attention to. And that means paying attention to the little things that you do well, the small efforts at kindness, the minutia of pleasure. You do this just because it's the healthy thing to do right now and not because you *feel like* paying attention to positives. If you pay attention to what you feel like paying attention to, you'll stay depressed. Besides, it's paying attention to the negative stuff about yourself that got you here to begin with. Staying depressed is easy; changing is hard. Take the road less traveled.

Love Detective

And what if you're the one always offering the reassurance? How can you navigate these treacherous waters? Well, there *is* something you can do to break the cycle. You can make a rule for yourself that you will refuse to give reassurance on demand, instead offering *unsolicited* reassurance spontaneously, randomly, and sincerely.

Here's what you could say when your ERS partner asks for reassurance the second time: "You already asked me that question, and I've already answered. I don't really want to get into that pattern of reassuring you and then you discounting or not believing what I say, because it makes me feel bad about myself and our relationship. Instead, let's try something new. I'm going to offer plenty of evidence of how much I love you, of how terrific I think you are. But those clues are going to crop up when you least expect them. I'd really appreciate it if you would try to find all the little clues that I give out, ways I'm telling you how much I care. That way, I won't get frustrated and dispirited, and you'll get real evidence of how I feel."

You can call this game "the love detective." Begin each morning by giving some unsolicited reassurance and then follow it up with random acts of kindness and words of encouragement. Keep track of the clues you leave hidden in plain sight and in the evening; match up accounts. Challenge yourself to make sure that your reassurance is very *specific* and *focused*. If you need a formula, use this one: "When you do X in situation Y, I feel Z." For example: "When you make the bed in the morning, I feel so taken care of." Or "when you smile that way, I can see a little piece of your soul that is so beautiful." Or "when you remember to take out the trash, I know how hard you're trying and I respect you so much for your efforts." Little things make all the difference. Noticing the little things, calling attention to them, magnifies them. The second rule of life is this: "whatever you focus on grows." The first rule of life is "if you can't make it better, at least don't make it worse." Little by little, step by step, things get better. If you're the depressed partner who falls into that ERS pattern, get yourself a little notebook and begin collecting hidden prizes. Your partner is going to surprise you, so don't let any of the clues go unnoticed or uncollected. Write them down when you find them so you can come back to them later. Keeping a log of reassurances will help you validate yourself and will give you material to use in offering appreciation. The voluntary exchange of appreciation is a wonderful way to tend the home fires and keep love glowing.

Depression and Aggression

Interestingly, many people who are depressed fall into a pattern of being shy and self-effacing with strangers but harsh and unkind to the people they love the most. They lash out verbally in the most unpleasant ways, only to feel guilt and shame later on but powerless to stop the behavior.

This is another catch-22 from depression hell. Some clinicians believe that depression is a kind of grieving, and that grieving goes through different stages. These include stages of protest, despair, and detachment. In this frame, "reassurance-seeking behaviors actively communicate despair and may be a form of protest ... [N]egative feedback-seeking may be a way of communicating either despair or despondency about the self [and] [a]ggression may either cause or result from emotional detachment (Katz and Joiner 2001, 139)). Emotional detachment is painful, and people who are in pain often lash out. Just as there is a complex dynamic at work in so many aspects of depression—the cognitive, the biological, and the social dimensions of experience—a blurry reciprocal connection also exists between depression and loss.

And even though we don't usually think of the "blessed event" of bringing home baby as a loss, it is—loss of the familiar, loss of freedom, loss of what was, loss of identity, and loss of a way of life. Desirable though it may be, transitions involve loss and parenthood is loss before it is gain. And for some people, loss is excruciatingly painful.

How do we manage pain? How do we manage anger? Pain and anger are universal human experiences, but we manage these basic human experiences differently. Some people are inclined to aggress. In their fury, they lash out at those around them and take steps to "even the score." Others tend to hold their anger in. They stew over perceived injustices without directly expressing their ire, or they attempt to ignore, minimize, or distract themselves from their anger. Still others orient themselves in a constructive direction. They draw on their anger to make changes for the better, such as opening lines of communication, resolving conflict, and setting things right. What accounts for these individual differences in anger-management strategies? What factors tip the balance, allowing people to make constructive, as opposed to destructive, use of their anger? The answer to this age-old question may lie partly in whether we experience shame or guilt (Tangney et al. 1996).

Shame and Guilt

Some people tend to use these two terms interchangeably, but shame and guilt are two very different experiences. Shame is a global feeling. Guilt is a very specific feeling. When we feel ashamed, we feel exposed, worthless, and powerless to cover ourselves, powerless to hide from critical and condemning eyes. Shame is crippling. Shame is so painful, global, and thorough that it offers no escape. Backed into a corner, the shamed person often responds by lashing out defensively, as if trying to force those critical, condemning eyes to look away. Only, the feelings of condemnation actually come from inside you, not "out there" in others. Guilt, on the other hand, alerts us to bad behavior and a need to repair relationships. Sociopathic people who exploit and harm others do so without shame but also without guilt. We need guilt because it is part of our social guidance system, alerting us to our need to change our ways and mend our social net. Guilt lets us take into account another person's perspective, and this is what makes the difference between lashing out or avoiding, on one hand, and constructive problem solving, on the other (Tangney et al. 1996).

The crushing, entrapping quality of shame can cause people to lash out (which damages relationships). It can also cause people to avoid problems and people (which also damages relationships). And shame can cause people to oscillate between lashing out and avoiding like a pendulum, swinging wildly between two equally damaging and unsatisfactory alternatives. But people who are depressed and who feel ashamed typically don't know *how* to do things differently, not at that moment anyway. If they could, they would.

Fredricka and Dion were like that. Fred was very successful in her career, and she enjoyed a vibrant social life. Getting pregnant came as a surprise. She wasn't really planning on getting married any time soon, but the pregnancy changed that. She was getting older and she didn't really believe in abortion, so she and Dion agreed to raise the baby together, see how things went, and then consider whether to marry. But Fred was surprised at how difficult she found motherhood. It wasn't the mothering, per se, that she found difficult; it was the loss of her former life and her former self that she couldn't quite get used to. Dion was supportive, but he was also ambivalent—happy to provide a check but preferring to wait until the baby was older and more interesting to really get involved. Fred felt like she had fallen into a great, bottomless chasm, and the more she hated how she felt, the more she lashed out at Dion. She angrily accused him of worthlessness, called him every name in the book, and imputed his motives and his intentions. And every time she did these things, she felt ashamed of herself. Fred didn't know how or when exactly she had become this monster, but she couldn't escape herself and she couldn't seem to change either.

Secrets of Successful Self-Regulation

If you are depressed, if you feel destructive shame more often than constructive guilt, if you find yourself caught in this terrible, horrible, no-good, very bad cycle, take heart. There is hope. In the last two decades, research psychologists have discovered several secrets of effective self-regulation. The key to managing emotions is to control where your mind goes, and this is a skill that is learned and perfected with rehearsal (Ayduk et al. 2000; Ayduk, Mischel, and Downey 2002; Eigsti et al. 2006).

It turns out that the quality we call willpower, controlling your feelings and actions in the face of frustration, temptation, rejection, and anxiety, is rooted in the ability to turn your mind away from a distressing situation, thought, or emotion and engage cooling thoughts instead. In the mid-1960s, psychologist Walter Mischel and his research team at Stanford University did a series of experiments to find out how children learn self-control in the face of temptation. Their subjects were four-year-olds at the Stanford day-care center who were shown a tray of delectable treats—marshmallows, cookies, candy, and so forth. The child was asked to choose a treat, and then the experimenter explained that he had to step out of the room for a few moments. But before he left the room he gave the child a challenge, telling her that if she could wait until he came back, she could have two of the treats instead of one; if she rang the bell to call him back sooner, she could have one but not two. A team of scientists then watched from behind a one-way mirror. With varying degrees of success, each child struggled to wait as time ticked away. The most successful kids were the ones who distracted themselves by singing, looking away, crawling under the table—basically doing whatever they could to take their mind off the agony of waiting and the tempting delight in front of them (Lehrer 2009; Mischel and Gilligan 1964).

When it comes to depression, the agony of waiting has to do with waiting to be noticed, reassured, or appreciated. The temptation is to imagine that by demanding reassurance or by accusing the ones you love of not paying enough attention, you'll be able to meet your needs and feel better. The temptation is to convince yourself that you can lash out and still create a loving home and have the kinds of warm, affirming, and supportive relationships that we all need and crave. Switching your thoughts so that you can wait, so you can tolerate the uncertainty and discomfort, so that you can choose the kinder words that are more likely to produce the long-term results you desire, is hard. Switching the focus of your thoughts, distracting yourself, is, of course, more difficult for some people than for others. The same is true of most everything in life—people are able to do different things with differing levels of ease. The good news is that *all* people can learn new strategies, even if this new learning happens to be difficult.

So when you find yourself feeling "hot," angry emotions, you will need to train yourself to cool down first before speaking or acting. One strategy that helps you get some distance on these moments is journaling. However, it's very important to fit your journal work into a specific format. You will need to use a format that helps you separate events, interpretations, feelings, and urges. These four items often get confused, and it's important to distinguish between them in order to see the situation clearly. Once you've identified the sequence behind the strong emotions, it will be important to carefully plan and structure your words and actions to get the results you want. This requires waiting. The desired response is the marshmallow (imagine you're one of those kids in the Stanford study). Remember: you get more of what you want if you wait. In his classic guide to negotiating with difficult people, *Getting Past No*, Harvard business professor William Ury recommends the strategy of "going to the balcony" to help cool hot emotions. The "balcony" is a metaphor for a mental attitude of detachment (Ury 1991). I like the acronym DOOR (as in, going to the DOOR), where D stands for detach, O for observe yourself, O for observe the other, and R for respond, don't react. It's tempting to imagine that reacting to your emotion will solve it; but in reality, just about any knee-jerk reaction will make a situation worse, while taking the time to respond might make things better. And the first rule of life is this: if you can't make it better, at least don't make it worse.

Postpartum Rituals of Transition

In all societies since the beginning of time, men and women have faced the task of becoming family. And throughout history, societies have devised rituals, customs, and traditions that helped people manage the anxieties of the transition and the ambiguities of parenting. In China, new mothers must "do the month," a time of physical restriction, rest, and pampering by female relatives. Twenty years ago, postpartum depression was unheard of in China and anthropologists attributed the relative ease with which new mothers transitioned as a function of the massive supports that women received in doing the month

(Pillsbury 1978). But times have changed. China is rapidly becoming more Westernized. A blizzard of social and economic changes has blanketed that nation, eroding time-honored customs and protective traditions. Today postpartum depression is as common in China as in any other modern industrialized country (Lee et al. 2001).

Perhaps we can begin to understand our moral obligation as a society to overcome our deeply held value of strident independence and, instead of medicating motherhood, begin to mobilize traditions of support for new parents. Perhaps we can begin to see ourselves as morally responsible for the well-being of others in our community and find ways to avert the perfect storm that is postpartum depression.

Exercises for Chapter 3

Exercise 1: Play the Love Detective Game

When it comes to reassurance, agree with your partner to only ask once. Instead of asking the second or third time, concentrate on your mission to find clues that you are loved. Then, every time you find one, mention it out loud and show your appreciation, or write it down in your notebook so you can be sure to mention it later Then pick your time carefully when you can express your appreciation with specific examples. Appreciation means so much more when it is unsolicited and when it is specific.

We all love to have our efforts noticed, and appreciation is a powerful lubricant in social relationships. Remember that when you're depressed you are more likely to seek and attend to negative information that confirms your worst fears. In order to turn this around, you have to intentionally seek and attend to positive information. You probably get plenty of evidence pointing in the other direction. In fact, you're both great and not so great. Try to be willing to be in the dissonance, opening yourself to the possibility that you might just be a mixture of good and bad like everyone else.

Here is a useful rule to live by: if you're going to criticize (yourself or anyone else), you must also be able to identify four or five positive things as well—but you only get to write down the positives. So, start keeping track of the positives in your notebook.

Exercise 2: Show Appreciation

Identify several ways that you already show appreciation:

1.

2.

3.

4.

5.

Identify some new ways you could show appreciation. You can always poll your friends for new ideas, and you can even go to www .surveymonkey.com and create a ten-item survey for free. E-mail the link to however many friends you want, and the survey monkey will tabulate your results. You can set it to be anonymous or not.

Show appreciation with words. Think of some general guidelines, but if you have or come across some really good specific compliments, then feel free to add those to your menu.

1.

2.

3.

Show appreciation with actions. I'm putting more room for notes under this category because I think that we tend to overuse words to the point where they become less meaningful. I want to challenge you to start thinking differently and outside the box. Of course, if you already use actions more than words, you'll do better to challenge yourself to generate more examples involving words.

1.

2.

3.

4.

Show appreciation with tokens, gifts, and symbolic gestures. Some people are very skilled at choosing cards and gifts (even small, inexpensive gifts) that show the receiver that they've been seen and noticed. It's an adult version of "peek-a-boo, I see you!"

1.

2.

3.

Show appreciation with affectionate gestures. It's very important that your affectionate gestures not carry an implicit demand for sex, especially if your relationship has gotten into a rut or if sex has been absent or conflicted for a while. If sex has become problematic, you'll want to time your gestures very carefully to happen on the fly, when you're running out the door, or in some other context in which sex is unlikely to follow.

1.

2.

3.

Exercise 3:
Expand Your World

Talk to one stranger every day—keep the focus on them. You want to focus on your new conversation partner to break out of your context. Pain draws your attention to yourself. Think about it: if you have a toothache, there's not much else you can think about until you get that pain to go away. But if you get distracted enough, absorbed in some other task or something outside of yourself, then the pain occupies less of your awareness. It's the same with emotional pain. And, while deliberately focusing on others when you're depressed pulls you out of yourself and distracts, it also expands your world by offering opportunities to be pleasantly surprised. Remember to journal in your notebook about these efforts and the results you get, only committing to paper the positives.

Exercise 4:
Tending to Relationships

Relationship	Plan of action	Results
Next-door neighbor	Say "hello" and initiate light conversation. Take a token (loaf of bread, garden basil, etc.).	Warm feelings

Figure 3.1: Relationship Improvement Worksheet

Working on your relationships can go a long way toward decreasing your feelings of isolation. For this exercise, you can do the work in your notebook, using the Relationship Improvement Worksheet as an example.

List three relationships you want to maintain and improve.

1.

2.

3.

Create a plan defining small steps toward enriching these relationships. You might start by thinking about whether the relationship is more rooted in words, actions, or symbolic gestures. Then write down the ways you have typically expressed appreciation alongside the ways each of these people expresses appreciation to you. You might just be surprised at how much appreciation people express to you that you overlook on a day-to-day basis.

Here's an example: Dorey is a friend I don't see very often anymore, and I know she leads a very busy life. She checks her e-mail several times a day because her job involves being at the computer a lot. Since she's not able to write long, drawn-out letters (and not inclined to read them), I just keep an eye out for random news articles, jokes, and tidbits that might be of interest to her and send them along. I occasionally (not too frequently) send short messages to her that I think she might be interested in, and she does the same for me. That way we keep in touch, and show that we "get" each other.

Follow through with implementing your plan in small steps. Keep the rate of contact comfortable—not too frequent but not few and far between either. One step a week might be enough if you have a clear plan and your steps are spelled out specifically.

After a few months, take stock of your results. Pay careful attention to positive results and take care to identify what you don't know. Accuracy in this evaluation is important because this situation may be ripe for misinterpretation (if you don't get a response right away or you get a confusing response), and you may be sorely tempted to fill in the blanks with speculation. If you really don't know, acknowledge that and keep working the plan.

Correct as necessary. Be careful not to correct by ramping up the volume, trying to get attention from someone who might be distracted, busy, uninterested, or burnt out. Instead, keep your focus on gentle efforts, subtle efforts consistently applied. When you get an overtly negative response or some specific feedback, take that feedback seriously and adjust your efforts accordingly. Always stop doing something that someone else says is rubbing them the wrong way, and respect the other person's boundaries.

List three relationships you need to repair, then repeat the above steps.

1.

2.

3.

As you pursue these plans, try to remember the first and second rules of life:

1. If you can't make it better, at least don't make it worse.

2. Whatever you focus on grows; focus on positives.

Exercise 5:
Shame Inoculation

Identify your shame buttons and cover them. The more familiar you are with the signature of your own emotions and the distortions that move you into shame, the more you will be "covered." In healthy relationships, each person gets to ask and each person gets to accept or decline requests. That means you get to say no, and it means you have to be prepared to manage your own disappointment when you are told no or asked to back off. Disappointment is a part of life; it is not a reason to feel ashamed.

Triggers for Shame (The actions or events that tend to lead to your feelings of shame)	Cognitive Distortions (The thoughts that hit after the trigger; what you tell yourself about the trigger that inspires shame)	Remedial Action (What can you do differently to help you avoid reacting to a trigger like this with shame?)
Making a mistake	I should know better.	Remind myself that I'm imperfect. Embrace the learning curve!

Figure 3.2: Shame-Inoculation Worksheet

Exercise 6:
Using Guilt as a Tool

Cultivate the capacity to listen to guilt as an alarm signaling you to take positive action to repair a relationship. Remember: reassurance seeking is not relationship repair.

Identify people in your life whom you admire for their relationship-repair skills and ask them to share their secrets with you. For instance, you might say something like:

"I've noticed that you're very good at [fill in the blank with a specific social skill]. What's your secret? What do you pay attention to about a person before you [fill in the blank with a specific interpersonal behavior]? If you were going to teach someone to do what you do, where would you start?"

Exercise 7:
Create Your Own Rituals

In keeping with your vision of a happy, healthy family life, create your own rituals. Rituals that you honor, enjoy, and treat as important will provide a structure to help you stay active and involved with others. *Simple Abundance* by Sarah Ban Breathnach offers many suggestions (Ban Breathnach 1995). Her book elaborates six principles that build upon each other: gratitude, simplicity, order, harmony, beauty, and joy. For example, she offers suggestions for developing habits to cultivate gratitude, habits to make doing routine tasks (like paying bills) a little bit more pleasant (and therefore less likely to be avoided), and many ways to mark holidays and the passage of time (transitions and seasons) with rituals.

Here's an idea: identify one holiday per season and create a plan for celebrating. The brain organizes memories in categories, and retrieving memories often depends on their distinctiveness. Since the change of seasons is distinctive in many places, many memories are filed with "tags" for different seasons. I think this is probably why I notice that people who have experienced deep personal losses often grieve when the seasons change—the change of seasons is associated with a whole new set of memories associated with the loss. This will be true for you, too, if you live in a part of the world where there are seasons and if having a baby has involved loss of aspects of lifestyle that were positive for you. So, deliberately creating ways to mark the transition from one season to another in pleasant ways can help you take charge of populating your memory banks with good feelings. Also, it will create loving memories for your children. With repetition, what starts out as just one instance becomes a habit. How will you celebrate spring? Summer? Fall? Winter? What kinds of associations do you want to have? What kinds of associations do you want your baby to grow up having? Write down several ideas for each season.

Here are some ways that I've created personal and special rituals for myself and my loved ones:

- For Halloween, I like to have people over to watch *Young Frankenstein* (1974). We also always carve a pumpkin and play scary music out the window for the trick-or-treaters. I chose Halloween to celebrate because it's always been special to me. I think it has something to teach all of us. It seems to me that the true meaning of the holiday is, "In life, you've got to face your fears in order to get the goodies." My daughter now remembers fall as a wonderful time of year when we changed the decorations in the house, bought pumpkins, and made her costume. And whenever she faces something new, a challenge or transition that she's afraid of and would rather avoid, she remembers the message of Halloween and faces her fears.

- Thanksgiving is different each year at my house—except the menu is pretty well set after nearly thirty years. At my house, we hate turkey carcass, so we've created a ritual of always making a turkey roulade with the dressing rolled inside. We had loads of fun (and a few memorable disasters) trying new recipes. And now Thanksgiving is associated with a spirit of adventure as well as gratitude. Try new recipes and each year and keep the ones that work.

♦ Another Thanksgiving idea is to create a ritual out of volunteering at the local homeless shelter or food bank on this day. With this ritual, children grow up with a sense of contributing to the larger community, and giving thanks becomes a way of giving beyond oneself.

♦ At Christmas I always host a tree-decorating party. Then, when I put away my decorations each year, I write out my goals (one could as easily call them wishes or prayers) for the next year. That way, when Christmas comes around again and I pull out the decorations, I can do a review and list what I'm grateful for. Each year the stories of Christmases past become richer. Every ornament has a past. The moments that once were difficult have become occasions for laughter, and that makes each new difficulty a little more bearable. When everything goes wrong we now remember to pause, laugh, and take note because today's fiasco will eventually be another funny story added to the tree.

♦ For New Year's, I like the concept of "reverse resolutions." Reverse resolutions go like this: make a list of everything you accomplished the year before. Voila! Now you have last year's resolutions and you've met every one of them!

Remember that almost every month has a holiday that you can celebrate in your own way. Or, if there isn't a formal holiday that appeals to you, go ahead and use your creativity to formalize your very own holiday. Celebrate whatever gives you joy! But remember, it is the repetitions that make a habit, so, if you're going to create something from scratch, you'll have to be intentional about repeating it each year. It will take several years before you'll really feel like you have a sense of continuity.

Exercise 8:
Connect to Community

If you don't belong to a distinct community or subculture, start looking for ways to find one. Many activities lend themselves to community, but the sense of community typically develops slowly over time as the same people gather year after year for some common purpose. Gradually you notice that you look forward to hearing the rest of someone's story; you miss their smile or their laugh. Little by little you come to recognize a fabric and to appreciate how each person contributes to that fabric. You gravitate toward some people more than others and begin to form friendships. One day you realize just how meaningful that friendship is to you.

What activities are you involved in where you might meet the same people over and over again? If you don't currently have any, where might you start? Think about the context of your life, the places you go regularly. Your sense of community might come from some apparently irrelevant source. Every spring I look forward to the opening of our local farmers' market. I've come to look forward to my weekly purchase of fresh fruits and vegetables. And there is a particular flower man and a certain soap lady whose smiles I look forward to seeing.

If you've moved around a lot and haven't had the opportunity to develop a sense of community, this could be a time to consider intentionally cultivating this particular feeling of connection. Online communities are a place to start for some people, but, ultimately, online relationships are not going to fill this essential need. But the Web can help you gather ideas about how to go about creating meaningful connections and community. Remember, this takes time and effort, so keep your goals modest and break your goals down into small steps so you can proceed slowly. Start with your existing routine. Open your eyes, notice, smile, greet. The people around you are part of a fabric, and you have an opportunity to expand your awareness of connection.

CHAPTER 4

Expectations Meet Reality: The Perfect Storm

It was the best of times; it was the worst of times.

Charles Dickens, *A Tale of Two Cities*

Most parents approach the birth or adoption of a baby with great anticipation and excitement. Their lives are about to change—forever! Most of the people I meet planned their pregnancies, whether they conceived before marriage or after. And in an age where abortion is a choice, most parents welcome the baby with open arms—this baby is *wanted*. But few parents are prepared for the emotional extremes they encounter when they come home with their bundle. All of them know that their life will change, but it's as impossible to anticipate what it will actually feel like as it would be to describe the taste of a banana to someone who has never eaten one. With the new baby, a tidal wave of changes rushes in upon the parents. As one father put it: "Think about how much you think your life is going to change, and now times it by ten" (Gianino 2008, 219).

Unexpected Changes

And just what are some of these changes? Consider this list: your priorities shift; your social life changes; you find yourself more isolated, with less time for other relationships just when you need the relationships most; you're exhausted; your body image is shot; you don't feel like having sex but you miss it (or you don't miss it but your partner does); you and your partner may have conflicting views about parenting; your roles are in flux around housework and child care; and you may struggle to balance high levels of emotional investment in both job and home life, but that balance is suddenly slippery (Gianino 2008; Barnett and Hyde 2001; Patterson 2000). These massive changes are not unique to biological parents; they also occur in adoptive families, whether straight or gay (Braun 2006; Alexander 2001; Lobaugh et al. 2006). In this chapter we'll examine the many stressors that a couple must face and the many changes they must make in order to successfully navigate the transition to parenthood. These changes are usually more easily imagined than lived, and they often clash with reality to create disappointment and conflict. By identifying predictable pitfalls, parents can develop a more clear understanding of what lies ahead.

A Convergence of Stressors

It should be apparent by now that, contrary to popular belief and modern mythology, postpartum depression does not strike from outside like a motorist blowing through a red light. Neither is postpartum depression like diabetes or heart disease. Rather, postpartum depression unfolds from within as the end product of a complex interplay of factors: unmet expectations (Fox, Bruce, and Combs-Orme 2000; Belsky 1985; Harwood, McLean, and Durkin 2007), habits of thought (Cutrona 1983; O'Hara, Rehm, and Campbell 1982; Liabsuetrakul, Vittayanont, and Pitanupong 2007), habits of relating (O'Hara, Rehm, and Campbell 1983; Sanford 2006; Figueiredo et al. 2008), sleep deprivation (Okun et al. 2009; Goyal, Gay, and Lee 2009; Medina, Lederhos, and Lillis 2009), and a culture that neglects to provide the level of support and mentoring that once existed to help people navigate life's transitions (Stemp, Turner, and Noh 1986; Becker and Lee 2002; Dennis and Ross 2006).

Hidden Expectations

When I was pregnant, if anyone had told me that I had expectations about what my baby would look like, I would have said, "Bah, humbug! All white babies look alike." Then Emily was born, and I found myself surprised. Well, guess what? It's impossible to be surprised or disappointed unless one has expectations—so, clearly I had expectations. I just didn't *know* that I had expectations, and I didn't know what they were. But when I held my baby with her full head of hair and found myself surprised, that's when I knew that the expectations had been there all along. I had expected her to look like my baby pictures—bald as bald can be. And the fact that I had expectations also came as a shock. Many of us try to avoid having expectations—at least as far as we're conscious of. But expectations are often held outside of awareness, and they are the cause of many rude surprises. As you might imagine, having expectations, especially unacknowledged ones, can be the ionic charge that sets the storm clouds of postpartum depression roiling (Cowan et al. 1985; Lawrence, Nylen, and Cobb 2007; Lawrence et al. 2008).

If you're still pregnant, ask yourself and your partner what you do expect. Try to be courageous enough to acknowledge your expectations, even if they seem outsized or unrealistic. Start talking about your expectations, trying as best you can to identify these hidden traps *before* the big event. If Scooter has already arrived, then start by listing all the little ways you've started to notice feeling surprised (or disappointed). Pull out your baby books and old photos if you have them and jot down some of the family stories you've heard about your babyhood. Were you laid-back or high-strung? Did you lie in an incubator for weeks or months before coming home? Were you born in another country and adopted? Collect as many stories as you can—whether you know it or not, some of these stories will probably inform your unconscious expectations. Next, take a look around you at your friends and family, the ones who have small kids. Reminisce about what you like and dislike about their parenting. Start asking the parents you know

about their surprises and disappointments. You might even go to www
.surveymonkey.com, make up a questionnaire with some of your questions, and e-mail it to the people in your circle of acquaintances.

Have fun sorting though all of this data and notice what comes up inside of you—assumptions about what causes what, for example, that lead you to imagine that if you just don't do a specific thing, then you won't have to deal with a certain unpleasant consequence. Above all, have compassion for yourself. "Perhaps underlying the capacity for surprise is a sense of humility. Surprise requires that one admit to not knowing everything and not thinking of every possible contingency—in short, to being human. Actively accommodating life experiences requires an admission of one's own vulnerability, of the inadequacy of one's preexisting meaning structures in the face of the challenges of reality, and of one's apparent smallness in the grand scheme of life" (King and Hicks 2007, 632). Life doesn't come with guarantees, and neither do babies. How do you cope with surprises? What about disappointments? How does your partner? Knowing your responses to life's curveballs will help you anticipate and create a plan for coping with the unexpected. As someone who's been there, I can tell you that a combination of structure and flexibility will be your greatest asset in the months ahead. Training yourself to look for the silver lining will also be important. The Spanish saying "No hay mal que por bien no venga" is roughly equivalent to the saying that every cloud has a silver lining—start noticing and collecting your own silver-lining stories.

A Well-Kept Secret

One of life's hidden expectations is the hope that relationship satisfaction will stay the same or increase with the addition of a baby. But the best-kept secret of marriage is that marital satisfaction declines over time. And the best-kept secret of parenthood is that marital satisfaction declines, often rather dramatically, after a baby is born (MacDermid, Huston, and McHale 1990; Doss et al. 2009; Kluwer and Johnson 2007). These findings have been replicated innumerable times; the knowledge is unquestioned among those who study or treat families (Schulz, Cowan, and Cowan 2006; Doss et al. 2009). Half of all divorces happen in the first seven years of marriage; one third happen in the first five years (Shapiro, Gottman, and Carrère 2000). For many of these divorces, the watershed event leading to the unraveling begins with (usually the wife's) declining marital satisfaction after the birth of the first baby (2000). The first baby brings a decrease in positive, affectionate interactions between husband and wife (or between partners in gay and lesbian families), an increase in conflict, and first a steep decline in the wife's satisfaction with and commitment to the marriage, then, sometime later, the husband's declining satisfaction (2000). Of course, couples who were unhappy to begin with are typically the hardest hit (Belsky 1985; Figueiredo et al. 2008). But happy couples are not immune.

Often the happiest couples are, paradoxically, the ones that suffer the greatest declines in marital satisfaction post-baby (Lawrence et al. 2008). Although we have known about and documented this drop for decades, it comes as a great shock and disappointment to many couples. And marital satisfaction will improve, after a time, for some of the heartiest and most skilled couples (usually once the child reaches school age), but some never recover (Lawrence et al. 2008; Doss et al. 2009). In today's society, most men and women becoming parents for the first time are virtually on their own when it comes to figuring out how to balance and address the needs of their new baby, their romantic partnership, and their commitments to work outside the family (Schulz, Cowan, and Cowan 2006). Relatively few couples—a mere 7 percent of women and 14 percent of men—remain stable or increase their marital satisfaction after the birth of a baby (Shapiro, Gottman, and Carrère 2000; Singley and Hynes 2005; Doss et al. 2009). Having a baby, whether it's the first or a subsequent child, is a major life stress. Parenthood changes the identities of individual men and women forever. It also changes their relationship, for better or for worse—forever (Barnett and Hyde 2001; Cowan et al. 1985). Given all these changes, how can we continue to return to the old theories of biological (and hormonal) determinism? If we do, we'll miss critical opportunities for prevention and intervention. But if we expand our understanding, we will also expand the scope of solutions.

Vulnerabilities, Stress, and Adaptation Interact

As we've seen, depression, like many other health conditions, is the product of complex interactions of factors in the biological, psychological, and interpersonal or social realms. Vulnerabilities combine with stress and are offset by protective adaptation factors (Demo and Cox 2000; Gage and Christensen 1991). Declining marital satisfaction, which sometimes leads to depression, also follows this path. Two of the *vulnerability factors* that have been studied extensively in relation to the declines in marital satisfaction that accompany the transition to parenthood are family of origin (conflict in the father's family of origin seems to matter the most) and a history of cohabiting (Doss et al. 2009; Cohan and Kleinbaum 2002). It may seem strange or even moralistic in our postmodern world to think of living together before marriage as a vulnerability factor; but over and over again, research has found that it is (Stanley, Rhoades, and Markman 2006; Stanley, Whitton, and Markman 2004; Tach and Halpern-Meekin 2009). Researchers have not quite figured out why cohabitating would be a vulnerability factor, but they speculate that it might indicate a level of ambivalence or a desire for guarantees in life that just don't hold up well to the realities of marriage and parenthood.

Stress factors include things like job demands, loneliness, and financial strain. One study found that giving birth at a time of relatively higher income and less financial stress could serve to buffer the couple against some of the stressors of birth (Doss et al. 2009). And finally, *adaptation factors* include things like communication skills and problem-solving abilities. Even for couples who have good skills and who functioned well as a couple before the birth, the months initiating them into parenthood come with increased negative communication and conflict—a time when problems seem much more intense, and confidence and dedication to the relationship typically suffers a hit (2009).

There are basically two schools of thought with regard to how stress affects people: one holds that stress brings out the worst in all of us; the other that stress only magnifies who we already are. And research suggests that both might be true—depending. The many changes that come with parenthood seem to magnify existing fault lines in habits of thought and habits of relating (Caspi and Moffitt 1991; Caspi 2000;

Caspi, Bem, and Elder 1989). Whatever skills one does have are certainly harder to access and put to use in the haze of sleeplessness, but it's also true that individuals who reported more problems with poor conflict management and problem intensity before birth showed significantly larger increases in these problems after birth (Kluwer and Johnson 2007). But the opposite was also true. The happiest couples were often vulnerable to suffering the steepest declines during this transition—possibly because couples who have the closest romantic connections find the transition to the tasks of parenting the most challenging, at least to the positive aspects of their relationships (Doss et al. 2009), or possibly because the happier couples tended to become pregnant the soonest (Lawrence, Nylen, and Cobb 2007; Lawrence et al. 2008). Either way, the data suggest that expecting a good relationship, a romantic relationship, to remain good in the same ways after baby might be a setup for a fall.

These patterns were not limited to heterosexual couples. Lesbians who conceived a child through artificial insemination evidenced decreases in love and increases in relationship conflict after the birth of their baby (Goldberg and Sayer 2006), and gay men who adopted also struggled to keep the relationship buoyant when negotiating the transition (Leung, Erich, and Kanenberg 2005). Taken together, these results suggest that the impact of the transition to parenthood may be especially potent when couples are at the extremes of both positive and negative relationship constructs (Doss et al. 2009). In other words, the happiest and the most distressed couples are the most at risk.

Expect the Best or Brace for the Worst?

I'm not providing you with all of this information about marital discord in order to make you feel afraid or hopeless. Certainly not. I believe that knowing the facts is empowering and can help you understand your situation more clearly. Knowing that most couples face difficulties after the birth of a child (contrary to the myth commonly purveyed in our culture) may let you off the hook a bit. It's not all your fault; this really is a hard time, and nearly everyone experiences it that way—whether they talk about it or not.

Fortunately, knowing what you're facing can help you prepare. If you or your partner is pregnant, or if you're about to adopt, you can discuss these realities and perhaps make a game plan for meeting them. If you're already in the thick of new parenthood, you can proceed from here with a greater clarity and less shame about your difficulties. But, should you expect that the worst will happen—that your relationship will go to hell in a handbasket, at least for a while—or should you expect the best?

We are currently enjoying a revival of positive thinking in our popular media with films and books like *The Secret* encouraging people to keep their hopes high and their thoughts positive (Byrne 2007). And maintaining positive expectations can be a good thing. Certainly, keeping thoughts positive *is* a good thing. But, since time immemorial, there has also been a cautionary undercurrent in the popular consciousness warning that high expectations could be dangerous, could be inadvertently setting us up for disappointment. Some recent research has finally shed some important light on the question by addressing the more nuanced question about when. When is it a good thing to keep expectations positive and when is it a better idea to keep expectations low enough to avoid risking disappointment? The answers might surprise you.

Which Strategy and When?

If you're the kind of charitable, forgiving, and optimistically inclined person who views your mate's most annoying habits and traits through a thick veil of love, if you give your mate the benefit of the doubt and put the most positive spin on his or her most annoying behavior, then positive expectations will likely do you a world of good. Positive attributions + positive expectations = more stable satisfaction over time (and less dissatisfaction post-baby). But if you are the charitable, forgiving, and optimistically inclined kind of person who also keeps expectations low, then positive attributions + negative expectations = steeper declines in marital satisfaction (McNulty and Karney 2004). Oops. Looks like if you're going to go to the trouble of having a sunny and forgiving disposition toward your partner's faults and mistakes, then trying to protect yourself from disappointment by keeping your expectations low might well backfire. The reasons for this are speculative but probably involve confirmation bias—the all-too-human tendency to filter what we experience by what we expect.

This tendency is so powerful and so profound that it can shape our very perception of physical reality. If you'd like to see a demonstration of this, go to YouTube (www.youtube.com) and search for "hollow mask illusion." You will find many video clips that demonstrate how a hollow mask, a mask that you know is concave, will appear convex as it slowly rotates. No matter how many times you look at the clip your brain will keep producing the illusion. You can also do a search for "confirmation bias" or "Pygmalion effect" and find interesting clips on experiments that demonstrate over and over again the power of expectations in determining what we actually experience from life or from others. But how does this confirmation bias play out in couples? To get a better idea, let's take a look at Jess.

Jess was one of those perpetually upbeat people who seemed to always wear a smile. Whenever he walked into a room, the mood of the whole group would lighten. Coworkers sought him out when they were down, and Jess's enthusiasm and encouragement would lift them up again. Until the divorce, that is. Finding out that his wife was cheating on him—had been cheating for quite some time and with different men—burst Jess's bubble and shook his world. Even after he got over the betrayal (or so he thought), even after coming out of depression and thoroughly processing his emotional experience in therapy, he still tended to brace himself inwardly—hoping for the best but secretly expecting the worst. At length, he did remarry and his old enthusiasm returned, lighting up his face and brightening the scene wherever he went. Except that he held back the deepest part of himself, and little by little the corrosive effect of self-protective skepticism began to eat away at his second chance.

Attributional style (our habitual ways of explaining why things happen) and expectancies interact to either magnify problems or buffer them. So, a positive attributional style coupled with positive expectations is the best way to approach life, yielding the most joy. But if you are a more pessimistic person, the kind who "keeps score" or raises an eyebrow and crosses your arms when your honey misbehaves, then keeping your expectations low will serve you well: negative attributions + negative expectancies = more stable levels of marital satisfaction during this stressful transition. These marriages are more stable but not necessarily as happy—after all, pessimism can tend to act as a self-fulfilling prophecy (McNulty and Karney 2004). In sum, which expectations are adaptive depends on the relationship context. When the relationship context is positive, positive expectations appear to be adaptive. When the relationship context is less positive, less positive expectations appear to be adaptive (McNulty and Karney 2004).

Which would you rather? A stable life of restrained happiness or to go for broke with a roll of the dice? These questions could be good food for thought or material for discussion. But be careful—sharing how you see your partner can be tricky business, especially if he or she is already depressed. But if you are depressed, or just inclined to protect your heart with pessimism, this could be a time to really reach down deep and make a choice. After all, you might not get to choose your circumstances, but you do get to choose your attitude.

Skills and Expectations

Attributions are not the only factors interacting with expectancies to predict stability or decline in the marriage after a baby arrives. Skills are also important. If you have oodles of relationship skills and negative expectations, you're likely to experience a steeper decline than if you have great relationship skills and boundless optimism. But if you're challenged in the relationship-skills department, then keeping expectations low is your very best bet for relationship stability (McNulty and Karney 2004). Jess had great skills, but once he lost that core optimism the very skills that were such an asset earlier in life became a liability. In order to turn his second marriage around and keep it from foundering on the rocks of negative expectations, he had to do some deep work and make some hard choices. He had to make the courageous choice to recognize his jadedness and embrace optimism in the face of uncertainty. It's hard to choose a positive attitude when you know you might get hurt—much harder than choosing to be positive by imagining that doing so will necessarily produce a great life. Life doesn't come with guarantees, and love, freely chosen, necessarily entails risk.

If, however, you are challenged in the relationship-skills department, then it might actually serve you well to keep your expectations low, a little closer to the ground. Although, in the research, couples who lacked relationship skills and had lower expectations also had lower overall marital-satisfaction ratings compared to the more skilled and optimistic couples, their marriages were very stable and were happy *enough*. Sometimes enough may be the most reasonable mark to shoot for (McNulty and Karney 2004).

Skills can be learned with intention, commitment, and repetition. Teaching relationship skills is beyond the scope of this book, but there are plenty of great resources out there that can be a real help. One that I highly recommend is *Fighting for Your Marriage: Positive Steps for Preventing Divorce and Preserving a Lasting Love* (Markman, Stanley, and Blumberg 2001). The authors are researchers at the University of Denver and have documented the effectiveness of their communications-training program over decades. Another is *Couple Skills* (McKay, Fanning, and Paleg 2006). Both of these books offer structured exercises to help you learn these important skills.

Gender and Roles: Expectations and Mythical Standards

The image of the involved father and the egalitarian marriage is very popular. Jean Twenge, documenting the changes in sex roles and expectations in her book *Generation Me*, writes: "GenMe women spend less time in housework than our mothers did; but we expect to split things fifty-fifty with our male partners, and when this doesn't happen we often explode. Or we do the work to avoid the fight, since we've fought about it so many times before, but are still steaming inside" (Twenge 2006, 196). We are bombarded by images of men and women defying traditional gender role stereotypes—men pushing strollers and women pounding gavels in courtrooms. We receive messages from the media and the culture at large that promise everything—we can have it all. But the emotional realities of juggling emotional, physical, social, and cultural logistics are not that simple. And research increasingly shows that violated expectations—the jarring discrepancies between what we think we're signing on for and what we get—account for a lot of this decline in marital satisfaction after the baby comes home (Grote and

Clark 2001; Goldberg and Perry-Jenkins 2004; Davis and Greenstein 2004). The culture has changed, and modern women expect both a fifty-fifty split in housework and emotional support from their partners. But the real-life behavior of most couples has not kept up. Today's men *are* doing more at home, but even doubling their contributions leaves them far from equally responsible in the domestic realm (Galinsky 2009; Harrington 2010). While it's true that black and Hispanic fathers may be more involved around the house and with their children, they are also significantly less likely to provide emotional support to their wives and partners (Fox, Bruce, and Combs-Orme 2000). Thus the disparity between women's expectations and men's behavior leaves many women disappointed and angry.

Conflicting expectations are hard on husbands too. Even though cultural expectations now demand that fathers contribute more to home caring and child care, fathers still feel the burden (perhaps self-imposed, perhaps externally imposed) to be the primary breadwinner. These new fathers are thus often caught in the crosscurrents of conflicting norms—to be fully engaged at work and to be fully engaged at home. This may be one reason why researchers are finding record levels of postpartum depression among dads (Fox, Bruce, and Combs-Orme 2000). Trying to do it all will drive anyone crazy.

Emerging Trends

There have been some positive changes happening on the economic front:

> In the 1970s, researchers noted that when a wife's income was greater than her husband's, the husband's role in the family was clearly threatened ... In the 1980s [researchers] found that the higher the wife's earnings relative to her husband's, the worse she said she felt about herself as a spouse. In 1996, 40 percent of white college-educated wives earned more than their husbands, as did 26 percent of all employed wives. And in these couples, wives' earnings relative to their husbands' had no marked effect on wives' marital experiences, only limited

effect on husbands', and generally positive effects on marital stability. (Barnett and Hyde 2001, 787)

But, even though today most couples have choices they didn't have or even imagine a century, a half century, or even a quarter century ago, sorting out roles is still a sticking point. "Having a baby suddenly means that you have little control over your life—the freedom to which you were accustomed vanishes, and your individual accomplishments are not as valued anymore. Parenthood has always been a difficult transition, but it's even more difficult for GenMe. When you're used to calling the shots, and then the baby dictates everything, it's hard to keep your sanity, much less get along with your spouse" (Twenge 2006, 94).

The daddy myth holds that men will do fully 50 percent of the housework, fathers will be equally engaged with the baby, and both mom and dad will balance high-powered careers and full-throttled parenting in perfect proportion. On some level of consciousness, fathers and mothers believe that the behavior of fathers will measure up to the myth. Usually, this is early in the parental game, before or just after the birth of the first child. In time, however, reality sets in, and on another level of consciousness it becomes apparent that mom is doing more than planned because dad is doing less than planned (LaRossa 1988). There is no such thing as 110 percent, much less two 100 percents. Perfect balance between work and home is an unattainable standard. Study after study reveals that gender roles drift toward traditional divisions of labor after a baby comes into the family. Among heterosexual couples, men still do less housework and spend less time with their children than women do (Greenstein 2000; Wall and Arnold 2007). This in spite of their intention to split household work fifty-fifty and despite their perception that they do successfully split housework and childcare fifty-fifty. The rub seems to be that while men are doing more than ever before, it's still not enough because women still bear the greater portion of the psychological burden (Galisnky 2009; Harrington 2010). What is also striking is the enormous variation in women's housework hours with transitions in birth compared to the flat and static average housework hours for men (Baxter, Hewitt, and Haynes 2008). Mothers of one child typically contribute 38 percent of the couple's outside-employment hours and 66 percent of the household work; mothers of two children typically contribute 22 percent of the employment hours and 70 percent or more of the household work (Sanchez and Thomson 1997). What is supposed to happen is not what actually happens.

The couple scrambles to uphold the myth, but the drift typically continues, often exacerbating the woman's discontent (Baxter, Hewitt, and Haynes 2008; Demo and Acock 1993; Gjerdingen and Center 2005). Moreover, once these unequal patterns are in place, it may be difficult to renegotiate them as the household structure changes later in the life course (Baxter, Hewitt, and Haynes 2008). Even gay and lesbian couples often struggle to keep from drifting into traditional "butch" and "fem" roles after a baby is born, particularly if one quits paid work to stay home in the full-time parent and homemaker role (Gianino 2008; Fulcher et al. 2006).

Power Determines Flexibility and Choice

I'm not arguing that women (or men) give up their expectations. Rather, I want to add some complexity to the idea of equal parenting. In most cases, at this point in history, parenting and home-caring duties aren't actually shared equally. And, in many cases, this can cause conflict between the partners. But not always. Because there are always exceptions to statistical averages, it behooves us to take a closer look at the gender divisions of home and child care in order to find out more about *what* works *when*.

Not all dual-income families are alike. In one study, couples were interviewed about their use of the Family and Medical Leave Act (FMLA) of 1993. This historic act gives workers the right to job-protected leaves of absence from work for family or medical reasons. The language of the law is gender neutral, covering men as well as women. Using the structure of the FMLA as a foundation for discussion, the researchers found that heterosexual couples tended to fall into two groups—those who had strong preferences about traditional versus egalitarian roles, and those who did not. Interestingly, for couples who didn't have a strong preference to start out with, practical and financial considerations determined the shape of their family work and parenting roles (Singley and Hynes 2005).

To see how this might play out, let's look at a couple from my own practice (their names have been changed). When she first married Riley, Blake thought she had effectively "settled" because he didn't match her in terms of economic and professional accomplishments. But when he gladly put his work aside to step into the traditional "wife" role, she discovered she had hit the jackpot. Their practical and financial considerations made this choice the logical one; the fact that Riley is competent at housework and child care and enjoys doing these things made the choice fly. Increasingly, many couples, like Riley and Blake, base the choice about who will stay home with the baby on these kinds of practical considerations—policies and benefits afforded by their employers (Singley and Hynes 2005).

Indeed, when researchers take a closer look at the career paths of men and women in so-called "dual-earner" families, three distinct groups emerge: high-status dual-career families, low-stress two-income families, and stratified families with a primary and secondary income (Barnett and Hyde 2001). Traditional gender roles work well in some families, and egalitarian roles work better for others. Which one works best depends on:

- How clear the expectations are ahead of time

- Whether expectations of one parent match those of the other

- How flexible the couple is when practical considerations upend original plans

- How much power each spouse has

In a Canadian study of men, specifically college-educated engineers employed in the energy industry, researcher Gillian Ranson found that the only men who challenged the demands and expectations of the workplace were those who had "arrived" in the sense that they, "by virtue of superior talent or possession of needed skills or simple seniority in an organization, had paid their dues and could therefore name their terms" (Ranson 2001, 22). This can be interpreted as these

men having power, and power is not often considered when researchers design studies looking at the division of labor question. Thus, we
really don't have a lot of information about how couples with low power
adjust differently than couples who have more power. Clearly, power
buys flexibility, and without flexibility, equality in work and household
is a fleeting aspiration for most couples—an elusive myth.

Traditional Women and Egalitarian Men

It's no surprise that a conflict would arise when a woman who
expects her husband to be very involved with housework and child care
finds herself in the traditional role drift. But another scenario exists
and has been well documented—one that is not as well known and not
as intuitively predictable. Some women actually like housework. Some
women actually like taking care of the kids. Some women actually love
the traditional role of wife and mom (Hackel and Ruble 1992). And for
some of these women, help from husband can feel uncomfortable—
encroaching, even.

Women who prefer traditional gender roles often feel disappointed
when their partner provides more help than they expected (Fox,
Bruce, and Combs-Orme 2000). And some men feel pushed aside—
not allowed to get involved as much as they would like (McHale et al.
2004). This maintenance of traditional role boundaries has been called
maternal gate keeping: "[b]riefly, maternal gate keeping is a collection
of beliefs and behaviors that ultimately inhibit a collaborative effort
between men and women in family work by limiting men's opportunities for learning and growing through caring for home and children" (Allen and Hawkins 1999, 200). Charlie and Payton are one such
couple. Charlie was supposed to be a tomboy. Her parents believed that
girlie girls were shaped by the toys they were given, so they provided
Charlie with androgynous toys—brightly colored blocks and rings and
genderless stuffed animals. But Charlie proved them wrong. Whenever
the other kids were playing hide-and-seek in the wooded park behind
their home, Charlie was playing house amid the clump of trees on the
far end. So when she and Payton got married and she became pregnant, Charlie was in her element. Saturday mornings were for cleaning

house; the pantry and laundry room were meticulously organized; and dinner was always hot on the table when Payton got home from work.

But Payton was raised by a single mom. He watched his mother struggle to pay the bills while still managing to shop, cook, do the laundry, and keep the house tidy (sort of). Payton learned to operate the washing machine when he was just five and had been getting dinner on the table for his mother's late nights at work since he was nine. Payton loved Charlie, and he was glad to see her so happy; but, in truth, he felt awkward and a little bit resentful seeing her take over the domestic domain with such panache. He didn't need to be instructed in how to fold towels (thank you very much!), nor did he think there was anything wrong with how he made lasagna (putting the casserole together with dry noodles keeps it from being too soupy). Payton is what some women would call an ideal partner—willing and even enthusiastic to take an equal role in keeping house. But, in this couple, Payton's efforts combined with Charlie's gatekeeping resulted in friction and unspoken resentment.

When one partner wants to be more involved in work that's not traditional for his or her role, perhaps it's best to go with this flow. If the more-traditional woman rejects her male partner's help, treats him like a subordinate, as though his standards are too low or he's simply not competent, then both partners are diminished (Goldberg and Perry-Jenkins 2004).

So, one of the first challenges a couple faces after bringing home baby involves sorting out the differences in what they expect of each other with regard to housework and child care and setting realistic expectations. At the end of this chapter I've included my idea for one way to sort these things out. I call it the housework game. It might be interesting to play the game two different ways—one way would be sorting for fairness, the other would be sorting for preferences. If you're *really* in sync and lucky, your results when sorting for fairness and preferences would be about the same. But whatever the ultimate choice in terms of family roles, the most important thing will be that each partner feels appreciated by the other (Allen and Hawkins 1999). Too often, as couples settle into a routine and become consumed by the business of life, they also begin to forget to say thank you, to remember that the little things make the biggest difference, and to look for evidence of love folded into the mundane. Maybe this isn't true for you; but just in case, I've also included some exercises and ideas to help you show appreciation at the end of this chapter.

Clock Time, Social Time, and Sacred Time

Dividing household duties and child-care responsibilities in a way that's comfortable (or at least workable) for each partner is very important to marital satisfaction, but it can be tricky. One of the complicating factors is the different ways we think about time and the proper ways to use it.

There are twenty-four hours in a day for all of us, but we each have different demands placed on us during that finite frame. Depending on our commitments—what we determine is really important—we'll spend those hours feeling harried and hurried, running like a gerbil on a wheel, or enjoying and savoring each and every moment, knowing that this moment will never come around again. "Our energy tends to become fully available for anything to which we are highly committed, and we often feel more energetic after having done it. We tend to find little energy for anything to which we are not highly committed, and doing these things leaves us feeling spent, drained, or exhausted" (Marks 1979, 31). Clock time is that finite, linear, nonreplenishable resource we all have exactly the same amount of. And the perception that we never have enough time, that sense of being frazzled and harried, comes not from a lack of clock time, but rather from our attitude and what we choose to commit to.

Commitments are socially constructed, and when we overlay socially constructed commitments on top of clock time, we get *social time*. When we have an attitude of scarcity, when we adhere to the illusion that we can do everything equally well, social time becomes a tyrant. Work demands commitment. Relationships demand commitment. Friendship networks, which are so essential for human health and happiness, also demand commitment. And whatever delicate balance of commitments you had achieved in life before the baby is challenged now by the reality of parenthood. Babies demand commitment.

Cultures differ in how they regard time, value time, and allocate it. Some cultures value all of human activity equally. Sociologists refer to these as *sacralizing* cultures (Marks 1979). Other cultures value some activities over others. Sociologists refer to these as *invidious* cultures (Marks 1979). Ours is an invidious culture. We are thus energized for some activities, the activities we find important, and we are drained by activities we find unimportant. When we find ourselves straining to fulfill various roles at work and at home and in community, the strain results from the fact that we are overcommitted to some activities, activities that our culture values more, and undercommitted to other activities, those that our culture values less and to which our culture accords less prestige (Marks 1977; Marks 1979). Drudgery cannot exist in a sacralizing culture because everything one does is equally valuable, equally worthy: "Involvement in multiple roles with multiple partners will not be experienced as overdemanding, as the social production of energy is at its maximum. People who are highly committed to all of their activities and partners will 'find' ample time and energy for all of them" (Marks 1979, 33).

Babies naturally live in sacralized time. They don't know from clock time or social time. Babies just *are*. Sometimes they're uncomfortable and they complain. Sometimes they are rapt, taking in the world—everything is new! Unless you are skilled at joining baby in the now, unless you are fascinated by baby's fascination with everything, it is very easy to begin to feel pressured into multitasking. Multitasking is the great modern myth, the lie that we in modern Western civilization have perpetrated on ourselves to give us the illusion that our worth is enhanced by something other than being fully present in the moment (Wicks 2010). In reality, multitasking fragments our experience and renders us hollow shells performing automatic tasks in a joyless existence. "Complaining that their lives have become if anything more hectic, new fathers and mothers report that sleep time, television time, communication time, sex time, and even bathroom time are all in short supply, thanks to their newborns. Paradoxically, they also say that they are more often bored. Sudden weight gains and soap opera addictions are commonly attributed to having too many idle moments" (LaRossa 1983, 579).

Babies are only babies once. This moment will never return. And though it may seem hard to enjoy the moment these days—when everything is changing and you're extremely busy but never seem to get "anything" done—consciously focusing on those small moments of joy that parenthood affords can really help. That's why multitasking can be so dangerous. Multitasking not only robs you of the moment, but it also increases cortisol and stress hormones and leads to a multitude of health risks, from dental cavities to heart disease (Wetherell, Hyland, and Harris 2004; Bosch, de Geus et al. 2003; Bosch, Turkenburg et al. 2003).

The opposite of multitasking is mindfulness. *Mindfulness* is simply being aware and present—mind, body, and spirit. We all know when we're interacting with someone who is distracted, and we all know it when someone is present to us. Babies sense whether we are present or distracted too. Sacralizing cultures practice mindfulness in one form or another, as well as some form of ritualized trance induction, usually related to worship: "Sociologically speaking, daily activities always take the form of routines that are patterned by cultural meanings, and these meanings are always typifications and expectations about reality; they are necessarily less rich than our full experience of the world. Periodic and regular ASC [altered states of consciousness] experiences allow people temporarily to step outside of their routine activities and to suspend the cultural meanings that 'rubricize' these activities. They are ventures from the known and familiar to the unknown and unfamiliar, and back to the known and familiar, which become progressively expanded by the process" (Marks 1979, 39). The people I know who have succeeded in cultivating an attitude of mindfulness are people who have developed definite habits for structuring some form of meditation, prayer, or worship (states that psychologists trained in hypnosis would call "trance" or "altered states of consciousness") into their lives.

The people I know who are most successful at being mindful (or seem to be, anyway) also develop strict mental boundaries and use compartmentalization to their advantage when needed. Compartmentalization is a necessary skill if one is to live mindfully—being present at each (or almost each) moment. In other words, if you're going to be present, you will have to be able to put other thoughts aside. This is what I refer to as *compartmentalizing*.

Amos had a wonderful ability to do this, and I asked him his secret. Amos was a graduate student who interned at the state mental hospital forty-five minutes out of town. He had developed a mental habit of checking himself on his drive home; if, when he arrived at a certain billboard, he was still thinking about work, he would make the deliberate decision to redirect his mind. What are your billboards, the signals you use to alert you that it's time to let go, to leave work behind and return to the present? Buddhist monasteries sound a gong at random intervals during the day to remind the monks to return to mindfulness, while Christian monasteries structure the day according to the medieval tradition of regular intervals of prayer that serve the same purpose. What reminders, either those that happen naturally or reminders that you construct into your day, can you use to remind yourself to return to the present?

Becoming the Happy Spouse and Parent

Marriage satisfaction declines dramatically for most couples once children arrive. The operative word is *most*. Most means "not all." It is possible to be one of the few for whom marital satisfaction remains stable or even increases over the transition to parenthood. Several keys to success emerge from the research literature. The first secret is attitude. Having an attitude of mindfulness, of deliberately choosing to be present even in the more routine aspects of housework and child care, is an attitude worth cultivating. Being intentional about keeping your thoughts positive is another. And in particular, keeping positive thoughts about your partner in the front of your mind is key.

In a longitudinal study of 130 newlyweds, researchers Shapiro, Gottman, and Carrère (2000) studied the experiences of individual mothers. They found that "what predicted the stable or increasing marital satisfaction of mothers were the husband's expression of fondness toward her, the husband's high awareness for her and their relationship, and her awareness for her husband and their relationship. In contrast, what predicted the decline in marital satisfaction of mothers were the husband's negativity toward his wife, the husband's disappointment in the marriage, or the husband or wife having described their lives as chaotic" (Shapiro, Gottman, and Carrère 2000, 59).

In other words, keep the love flowing. Maintain some semblance of order. Keep communications positive. Edit out the snark. In his study of gay adoptive couples, Mark Gianino noted that "some couples balanced the demands of caretaking and breadwinner roles with the adoption of a sanguine attitude to do the best they could as often as they could" (Gianino 2008, 229). The best you can as often as you can—no more.

The second secret is skills—skills to resolve problems, manage emotions, realign priorities, to keep communicating and to keep communications positive. Also helpful are skills to create and maintain a level of organization sufficient to keep a satisfactory level of consistency and predictability to life without degenerating into chaos, the hallmark of a hectic, invidious lifestyle.

Developmental psychologists studying the evolution of human personality over the lifespan talk about *ego maturity* as the desirable outcome of a life well lived. Ego development or maturity involves an ever-increasing ability to tolerate life's inconsistencies gracefully—the ability to be open and compassionate, connected yet separate: "People at the higher stages of ego development recognize that life's lessons are contextualized and that life's big questions may have a variety of valid answers. Ego development involves an increasing capacity to recognize conflict and experience ambivalence" (King and Hicks 2007, 629). This is very similar to Abraham Maslow's idea of self-actualization. Maturity necessarily begins with self-acceptance (Maslow 1962). Self-actualization goes on to balance spontaneity and control—the capacity to love and work and play tempered by self-restraint. The transition to parenthood is an opportunity for growth and an adventure in learning:

> Growth has not only rewards and pleasures but also many intrinsic pains and always will have. Each step forward is a step into the unfamiliar and is possibly dangerous. It also means giving up something familiar and good and satisfying. It frequently means a parting and a separation, even a kind of death prior to rebirth, with consequent nostalgia, fear, loneliness, and mourning. It also often means giving up a simpler and easier and less effortful life in exchange for a more demanding, more responsible, more difficult life. (Maslow 1962, 190)

All learning curves necessarily involve failure and frustration. But with hard work and commitment, with the passion necessary to be honest with yourself and with each other about what is truly important, and with clear-eyed expectations, it *is* possible to meet the challenges of becoming a family in today's world. Although there will necessarily be disappointments as well as frustrations, the pleasures of parenthood are innumerable. How can you anticipate what the sight of your baby's first smile will feel like or the sense of pleasure that runs through you when you decipher those first words? The decline in marital satisfaction is a well-kept secret because it is a statistical reality and by no means a given, and because even when marital satisfaction does decline, most people feel that the shift to finding satisfaction in family life is well worth it.

Exercises for Chapter 4

Exercise 1: Strategies for Identifying Your Influence

Most of us, but particularly those of us who hold to high standards, often confuse influence and control and become anxious whenever we do not get the results we want or need when the outcome is important to us. So let's begin by sorting for different levels of influence. We'll start with the easy thing first.

Identify seven things you definitely can control:

    1. My own thoughts—on a good day, if I put my mind to it.

    2.

    3.

    4.

    5.

    6.

    7.

What are seven things you definitely *cannot* control?

    1. The economy

    2. The weather

    3. Whether some else responds to my request, even when the request is reasonable

4.

5.

6.

7.

Identify seven things you can *influence* but not control:

1. The election—by voting, canvassing, and getting involved

2. Someone else's behavior, for instance, by asking nicely for what I need

3.

4.

5.

6.

7.

Identify seven things you don't know whether you can or cannot control:

1. My own thoughts when I'm ruminating

2.

3.

4.

5.

6.

7.

Now consider your ratings with these facts in mind: if another person is involved, you're never more than 50 percent of the equation. Even your own behavior and choices can be derailed by unforeseen circumstances beyond your control. This is why in some cultures people regularly state their intentions followed by some qualifier that basically conveys "if God is willing." This overtly acknowledges the limits of human agency.

Exercise 2:
Minimizing Ambiguity

As you know from chapter 2, people who get depressed tend to engage in certain habits of thought. One of these is a real discomfort with not knowing and feeling an intense need to have some idea of what's going to happen and when.

Babies play havoc with your ability to plan and are forever disrupting your illusions of control, which can be very challenging for some (if not most) people. This exercise will help you get a better handle on all the new unknowns in your life. You still may feel at sea much of the time, but exerting some effort here will help rein in the irrational "shoulds."

Create an action plan for those things you *can* control and would *like* to control but do not control yet. For instance:

1. I can be in control of getting the laundry done (but not when). I need to make a definite commitment to myself to throw a load in whenever I see an opportunity.

2. I can be in control of balancing my checkbook (but not when). If I commit to doing it the next time the baby naps, I might actually achieve some sense of order in dealing with my finances.

Streamline daily tasks. For instance, identify predictable sequences and follow through on some reliably:

1. I get out of bed, turn around, tuck in the sheet, fold the duvet, and prop up the pillows.

2. I go to the bathroom.

3. Finally, I go into the kitchen to get my coffee.

Create daily rhythms and routines and list them:
Every day after doing the sequence listed above, I spend at least fifteen minutes in silent, emptying meditation *before* going over my mental to-do list.
Here are some of my suggestions:

*   Begin the day with curiosity.

*   Establish a moment of silence and centering around midday.

*   Establish a routine for unwinding and identifying positives before bedtime.

Make a habit of writing down all your positive accomplishments and gratitudes, no matter how small. This will help you develop a habit of turning your mind away from negatives, away from the "I don't wanna hafta" narrative and toward optimism and opportunities for joy and gratitude.

Exercise 3:
The Housework Game

Because housework can be such a flashpoint for conflict and feelings of frustration as a new parent, I've created this game to help you get a better practical and emotional handle on the issue.

Getting Set

1. Buy a pack of multicolored index cards. You will need five or six colors. If you can't find a pack that has enough colors, you can make your own out of construction paper.

2. Divide up the cards by color. You'll be using a different color for daily, weekly, monthly, quarterly, biyearly, and once-a-year tasks.

3. Write one task per card. In the upper right-hand corner of the card, give the task an estimated time value that you and your partner can agree on. Some couples use 1 to represent a fifteen-minute unit, 2 for a thirty-minute unit of time, and so forth.

4. Once you have identified all the tasks involved in maintaining your household and your lifestyle, divvy up the cards between the two of you. If you both work outside the home, then you will probably want to divide the household tasks evenly. If one works part time and the other full time, then you will probably want a proportional division of household labor. If one stays home and the tasks add up to more than a full-time, forty-hour-a-week job (as I suspect they will if you do this exercise honestly and thoroughly), then the stay-at-home parent will have some tasks but not all. Divide up the spillover tasks in a way that seems equitable and fair to you.

Rules of the Game

Each partner has responsibility for the tasks they are assigned and may not supervise or comment on the timeliness or performance of the other, except during couple's meetings.

Hold a couple's meeting once a week (the same meeting in which you update one another on financial matters is usually workable). During this meeting, you can hold your partner accountable for how he or she performed his or her household tasks. Remember to always lead and end with positive feedback. Sandwich complaints between the positives in very specific language using the X-Y-Z format: "When you did X in situation Y, I felt Z." Be specific and limit emotion words.

Renegotiate tasks and expectations as needed.

CHAPTER 5

Getting Some: Sleep and Sex After the Baby

People who say they sleep like a baby usually don't have one.

Leo J. Burke

When we consider all the complex emotional and mental tasks that new parents take on and must negotiate in order to successfully make the transition, it's hard to imagine that sleep deprivation doesn't play a key role. And when we consider how the sleep deprivation that normally accompanies parenthood affects mood and ability to process information, regulate emotions, think flexibly, and solve problems creatively, it can hardly come as a surprise that marital quality declines. The arrival of a baby requires that new parents renegotiate their household strategies, rebalance family and work priorities, and set different boundaries with family and friends (Anderson and Sabatelli 2003). On top of all this, the partners also have to figure out how to meet the baby's needs, the needs of their spouse, and their own needs (Cowan and Cowan 1995).

Sleep, or rather the absence of sleep, turns out to be tremendously important in the development of depression. It might well be one of the main reasons new parents in our culture get depressed so often, given all the competing demands on our time. According to researchers Anna Marie Medina, Crystal Lederhos, and Teresa Lillis (2009), managing these multiple demands effectively and regulating the emotions that arise during efforts to cope with stressors requires precisely those cognitive skills most affected by sleep disturbance:

- **Verbal fluency**: Communicating needs and goals effectively

- **Sustained attention**: Focusing on a particular issue or goal

- **Working memory**: Juggling multiple goals

- **Cognitive flexibility**: Being able to see the situation from various points of view

Sex, like sleep, remains largely a mystery despite all that we know about it and discuss it. Sexual desire may be one of the most intriguing aspects of being human, a dimension that defies pinning down into convenient formulas or tidy little boxes fit for manipulation (Morof et al. 2003). When sex is happening in a marriage, when it's functional and pleasurable, when sex is "good enough," it accounts for about 15 to 20 percent of marital satisfaction (McCarthy and McCarthy 2003). But when sex is absent from a marriage or when it is conflicted, it becomes disproportionately important, accounting for up to 70 percent of marital unhappiness (McCarthy and McCarthy 2003). With the baby comes sleep deprivation and with sleep deprivation a couple's sexuality takes a hit. So with sleep deprivation affecting couple sexuality and marital happiness, can it be any wonder that some parents would become depressed?

The Effects of Sleep Deprivation

Let's take a peek into the lives of one very typical couple and ask ourselves whether hormones really tell the story: Dana and Kim never really knew what to expect from parenthood and never really knew what hit them. But after Parker came into their lives, nothing was ever quite the same. Some things were different and better—they seemed to be more attentive to each other now that they were in this together.

And they shared an uncanny ability to intuit when the other was flagging and step in. But some things were different and not so great.

Sleep was one of those things. Dana never was one to stay up late, pull all-nighters in school, or party until all hours. Plus she was raised by the kind of parents who really believed that whatever happens in life is up to you—good or bad, you make life happen. For Dana, that attitude translated into blame. No matter what, she felt that she was to blame. No matter how much Kim tried to reassure her or smooth things over with her laid-back attitude, Dana felt responsible—for everything.

So, when they got Parker, Dana's brain went into overdrive. When she lay down to sleep, her mama ears were on the highest setting. Heck, she was so alert that she could practically hear the potted plants grow. And try as she might, she couldn't figure out how to turn it off. Nothing anyone could say would convince her that she didn't carry total responsibility for Parker's welfare. She went through all the possible scenarios for sudden infant death, convinced that she was responsible for making sure that kind of tragedy didn't happen to her. The only problem was, she never felt she knew what to do or when enough was enough. It was as if she was in charge of making sure the world didn't blow up, but she couldn't figure out what to do or not to do with the red button. And, to Dana, *everything* looked like the red button. Everything seemed too important.

In fact, Dana and Kim were struggling with the effects of sleep deprivation, which transformed Dana's usual attentiveness into hyper-attentiveness and made it even harder for her to sleep. And so, with Parker's arrival, Dana began a vicious circle that would eventually spiral into depression. Interestingly, Dana and Kim are adoptive parents, and fully 15 percent of adoptive mothers experience postpartum depression—a figure statistically indistinguishable from the depression rate among birth mothers and not too very far from the depression rate for dads (Senecky et al. 2009).

While we all know that sleep deprivation will make us loopy, scientists have only recently begun to understand just how much sleep deprivation affects us and in what particular ways. But before we examine the specific impact of sleep deprivation, let's review some of the fundamentals of normal sleep.

Sleep Basics

Why do we sleep? This question has been asked since time immemorial and, to date, we don't have a clear answer. But we do have the answers to some related questions. For instance, if we ask what and how questions about sleep, then we get some very interesting information.

Normal sleep is characterized by alternating cycles of REM sleep and non-REM sleep. *REM* of course refers to rapid eye movements. One of the very first things that early sleep researchers noticed was that there are times when the eyes appear to be darting from side to side under the closed eyelids of a sleeper (Knott, Gibbs, and Henry 1942; Goodenough et al. 1959). REM sleep is when dreaming occurs. For many years, researchers were intrigued by (or one might say sidetracked by) questions about the meaning of dreams, an unanswerable question that now seems largely irrelevant (Beaulieu-Provost, Charneau Simard, and Zadra 2009).

Lately, the role of non-REM sleep has gotten research attention (Landsness et al. 2009). The slow-wave sleep that characterizes such nondreaming states is divided into four substages, creatively named stages one, two, three, and four. Each stage is progressively deeper (Walker and van der Helm 2009; Thase 2006). During the normal course of a night's sleep, non-REM sleep alternates with REM sleep roughly every ninety minutes or so (2009; 2006). The ratio of REM to non-REM sleep changes over the course of the night, so that stages three and four, the deepest stages of slow-wave sleep, predominate early on and the lighter stages (stages 1 and 2) predominate closer to morning (Walker and van der Helm 2009).

As we age, we lose slow-wave sleep (Thase 2006). Women tend to have more deep sleep or slow-wave sleep than do men, and men tend to lose slow-wave sleep earlier than women (2006). And, as the brain goes through all these electrical changes, it also goes through neurochemical changes. After all, chemistry is electricity when it comes to the brain (Walker and van der Helm 2009). Although these phenomena have been described with increasing precision, researchers are just beginning to figure out what they mean (Walker and van der Helm 2009; Walker 2009; (Siegel 2009). During the cycles of REM and deep sleep the brain appears to be carrying out something analogous to a computer's defrag program in a complex and elegant mechanism for consolidating memory and maintaining emotional equilibrium.

Functions of Sleep

The elaborate interplay of REM and deep sleep is apparently necessary for both remembering *and* forgetting—remembering facts and forgetting unpleasant emotions (Walker and van der Helm 2009). It now seems that REM sleep is the process the brain uses to *consolidate*: to organize and store facts as memories while deconstructing and parsing emotions from memories (Riemann, Kloepfer, and Berger 2009; Walker and van der Helm 2009).

You might have noticed that you can more easily remember emotionally charged experiences than emotionally neutral events. Take for example last April twenty-third—what exactly were you doing? You can't remember. You can't remember, that is, unless April twenty-third is an important date for you, a date that has emotionally charged memories associated with it. If April twenty-third is the anniversary of something particularly joyful, tragic, or even just distinctive, then you may well remember that date. In fact, laboratory research shows that good-quality sleep helps humans overcome learned fear responses, the fear we associate with intensely negative experiences (Pace-Schott et al. 2009). Thus the brain is prewired to heal itself from unpleasant, fearful memories and associations—if only we can get good sleep.

Unfortunately, one of the most prominent symptoms of depression is insomnia, although not everyone who gets depressed has this symptom. And, in turn, sleep deprivation exacerbates depression: it selectively impairs memory so it cannot retain positive and neutral events (Walker 2009; Walker and van der Helm 2009).

Sleep and Depression

The sleep patterns of depressed people thus have a distinctive signature. In the jargon of the trade, depressed people have a shortened REM *latency*, meaning that they go into REM sleep much too soon, sooner than do nondepressed people (Berger, VanCalker, and Riemann 2003). They also have more REM *density* than do normal people (2003). This suggests that whatever the brain does during REM sleep, it is doing it faster and more furiously in depressed people than it would otherwise. So, it would seem that people who are depressed are processing a whole host of emotions and trying valiantly to unhook feelings from events, but to little avail. They also have less deep, slow-wave sleep, the kind of sleep essential to the brain's ability to integrate isolated memories into general knowledge and necessary for creative problem solving and flexible thinking. It is the disruption of this integrative function that may well be behind the emotional reactivity, that tendency to have a hair trigger for intense emotional responses that we experience when we're operating on too little sleep.

Furthermore our ability to *modulate* our emotional experience depends on the connections between the emotional centers of the brain, like the limbic system and the amygdala, and the thinking, rational, parts of the brain, namely the prefrontal cortex (Walker 2009). The prefrontal cortex is the same part of the brain that is thicker in Zen masters and people who have a longstanding history of trance or meditation (Lazar et al. 2005). A depressed person gets less sleep, and, in turn, sleep deprivation disrupts these important connections.

Sleep Quality and PPD

Sleep and depression are linked in a host of ways. We've seen that depression can cause sleep deprivation or insomnia. The reverse is also true—sleep deprivation can cause depression (VanMoffaert 1994). Also, people who have depression with sleep disturbance tend to have worse symptoms of depression than do people who have depression without sleep disturbance. And the symptom most associated with recurrence of depression in someone who has already had one or more episodes of major depression, is—you guessed it—sleep disturbance (Abad and Guilleminault 2005). In fact, any sleep disturbance that persists for more than two weeks creates a significant risk for depression (Abad and Guilleminault 2005; Muzet 2005). And what do we know about bringing home a new baby? Sleep deprivation comes with the territory.

Sleep deprivation is guaranteed, whether the baby is born by vaginal birth, delivered by C-section, or brought into the family by adoption. Interestingly, women who go into labor during the night (and therefore have little or no sleep by the time the baby arrives) have a higher risk of developing depression (Billiard et al. 1994).

Some of this new-baby sleep deprivation is related to hormonal changes, but, as we've seen earlier in the book, those changes can be a result of a number of factors (the drop in hormones after giving birth; the hormones associated with couvade; the drop in testosterone and rise in cortisol experienced by some men after their partner gives birth; or the stress hormones that come flooding in with any big change, including adoption). And the direction of causation—or which caused what—is not always clear. While many people have speculated that a woman's sensitivity to her reproductive hormones might lead to sleep disturbance, the research suggests not: "The sleep regulatory mechanism is not substantially affected by the menstrual cycle" (Dzaja et al. 2005).

First-time mothers in one study were much more likely to become depressed if the baby had sleep problems, but not if the moms had good sleep *quality* (Medina, Lederhos, and Lillis 2009). And good-quality sleep means going to sleep quickly and easily. Among new parents, the most relevant and important risk factor for depression may well be having trouble falling asleep even when tired (Gay, Lee, and Lee 2004; Goyal, Gay, and Lee 2007; Goyal, Gay, and Lee 2009). In fact, sleep disturbance was a better predictor of recurring postpartum depression than age, race, marital status, or income level (Okun et al. 2009).

The Perils of Rumination

Rumination is a huge risk factor for depression (Nelson and Harvey 2003). For anyone, anywhere, ruminating—brooding and endlessly asking questions that do not lead to concrete action or solutions— poses a risk for depression. This is partly because rumination delays falling asleep and also produces fitful sleep (remember the signature of depressed sleep: short REM latency and increased REM density). This brings to mind a conviction that I hold but can't yet prove: As our culture moves further toward the invidious and away from the sacrilizing, as we become aware of so much more information while losing awareness of what we can and cannot control, rumination will become more and more common. We'll have to wait for anthropologists to study cognitive styles and coping styles in isolated, non-Western cultures before we'll really know if I'm right. And of course there are plenty of other aspects of modern life that interfere with sleep besides worry.

Looking for Help: Pills or Skills?

Trouble falling asleep can often be helped a great deal by learning how to turn off that terrible, horrible, no-good, very bad habit of rumination. But many antidepressants and sleep meds can make matters worse. Most antidepressant medications interfere with REM sleep; in fact, some theorists think that the antidepressant effect might largely come from this suppression of REM sleep since depression is associated with too much REM too soon (Thase 2006; LeBon 2005). Among currently available antidepressants there are precious few that don't suppress REM sleep. These are: trazodone (Desyrel), bupropion (Wellbutrin), and nefazodone (Serzone) fourth compound. There is also trimipramine (Rhotrimine), which is a weaker REM suppressor (Thase 2006).

Some antidepressants bring on REM sleep sooner instead of delaying the start of REM, and some reduce instead of increasing slow-wave sleep—oops (LeBon 2005; Gursky and Krahn 2000). In contrast to the reliable effects of antidepressants on REM sleep and, to a lesser extent, a person's ability to initiate and maintain sleep, antidepressant medications do not reliably increase slow-wave sleep (Thase 2006). One study followed fifty-one women from pregnancy, through birth, to several months post-delivery. These women had a history of postpartum mood disorder, and the researchers were looking for factors that might predict the recurrence of depression. Some of these subjects were given an antidepressant preventatively. But the antidepressant did *not* prevent sleep disturbance, and did not prevent depression from recurring if sleep was disturbed (Okun et al. 2009).

Fighting Depression with Better Sleep

So, if antidepressants aren't the answer to improving your sleep and fending off depression, what does help? Well, in fact you can get better quality sleep and more of it through two approaches that don't involve medicating yourself. These nonchemical approaches have been well studied and found to be helpful. The first sets the stage for the other: sleep hygiene and cognitive behavioral therapy.

Sleep Hygiene

Sleep hygiene has to do with how you organize life and set up basic bedtime habits, practices that facilitate going to sleep and sleeping well. You can Google "sleep hygiene" and pull up any number of sites with tips for creating good sleep-hygiene habits, including the tip sheet from the American Academy of Sleep Medicine and sleepeducation .com. But the principles are basic: create ritual and routines that will remain constant enough to train your brain to expect that sleep is to occur, and, beginning four to six hours before bedtime, avoid things that will have a stimulating effect.

Television, for example, tends to stimulate rather than truly relax. Television programming is meant to be engaging, and it's often difficult to unhook from the thoughts and emotions that TV sets in motion. Alcohol also has a stimulating effect once the immediate effects wear off. So, while a drink before bedtime might make you sleepy, it is also likely to lead to those 3:00 a.m. awakenings that so fragment the night and can lead to depression. Caffeine, of course, also has a stimulating effect. Beyond avoiding these, make sure your exercise routine happens earlier in the day—a good six hours before bedtime. And start to practice some kind of meditation ritual in the evening that relaxes you and helps you focus your mind away from problems.

Cognitive Behavioral Therapy

The other nonchemical approach that has been well studied and found to definitely be helpful is *cognitive behavioral therapy* (CBT) for

147

insomnia. Beyond explicit attention to sleep hygiene, cognitive behavioral therapy for insomnia utilizes stimulus control and arousal-reduction techniques (Thase 2006). *Stimulus control* refers to associating a behavior to a cue—whenever the cue occurs, the behavior follows. For example, your head hitting the pillow can become your cue. The behavior, which in this case is sleep, soon follows. *Arousal reduction* refers to the many ways we can reduce autonomic or emotional arousal.

While I was writing this book, I attended a conference on hypnosis and sat next to a physician colleague. We got to talking, and I became curious about his take on getting better sleep. I knew he had experienced the trials of sleep deprivation during his medical training, that he was a parent, and that he knew about hypnosis, so I asked him to share his pearls of wisdom. Joe told me that his daughter was born while he was a resident and he was on call a lot. Since his work was so demanding, it fell to his wife to take care of the baby and wake up when she cried. One morning he apologized for how disruptive his work must be to her since the phone had rung three different times between midnight and five o'clock in the morning. What really astounded him was that his wife never once heard the phone ring. Her mama ears were tuned to the baby crying but not at all to the telephone. That's when he decided that, since she had worked out a way to sleep through his on-call rings, he could darned well do the same—allow himself to sleep through the baby's noises without waking and without being bothered by the crying. So whenever he finished taking a call, as he walked back into the bedroom, he would touch the side of door frame as his silent reminder to turn his brain off and go to sleep (this is an example of stimulus control). Joe trained himself, using what amounts to self-hypnosis, to fall asleep as soon as his head hit the pillow, and his brain never again heard the baby cry during the night.

Cognitive behavioral techniques are at least as effective as are medications—at least and perhaps more so (Thase 2006). Besides being effective, cognitive behavioral techniques come without side effects, are not habit forming, and don't poop out over time the way meds can. Taking the short course around distress might get you feeling better quicker, but in the long run, the quick fix can end up costing much more. The potentially greatest advantage of CBT is evident over time, however, as effectiveness is more durable than drug therapy and benefits persist after therapy is terminated. So, even though CBT may be a more costly approach than pharmacotherapy in the short run, it becomes a cost-effective approach across six months or longer (Thase 2006). Americans tend to like the convenience of things that give us instant results, but the British would say using sleeping medications instead of CBT is "penny wise and pound foolish."

If you find yourself in a pickle like Dana did, there is absolutely nothing wrong and everything right about going on meds or even checking into a hospital until you get on track again. But the side effects and disruption these options can bring mean that it would benefit you to be proactive—to practice good sleep hygiene and learn how to be a good sleeper before you get into trouble. The long-term benefits of learning to be a good sleeper are also a really good reason to start teaching your baby good sleep habits right from the start. Good habits, started early, can save you from a world of hurting.

Breastfeeding

New parents should also know that breastfeeding increases deep sleep, slow-wave sleep in lactating women (Blyton, Sullivan, and Edwards 2002). Many parents start to supplement breast milk with formula at around three months with the idea that it will increase the baby's time asleep, helping the infant (and therefore the parents) to sleep through the night sooner. But studies show that the opposite might be true—that mothers and fathers of babies who breastfeed or are given breast milk at night get an average of forty-five minutes more sleep per night than do the parents of babies who are given formula in the evening or at night (Doan et al. 2007). Remember, of course, that statistics predict for a population, not for the individual, so there are no guarantees as to what will happen in your family.

To Nap or Not to Nap

One of the tips that you'll find mentioned repeatedly on all of these sleep-hygiene websites is an admonition against napping, particularly late in the afternoon. Is this same advice applicable to parents with infants who are struggling against sleep deprivation and trying to keep depression at bay? It is true that long naps and naps taken later in the afternoon can backfire, disrupting circadian rhythms and making it more difficult to get to sleep that night (Swain et al. 1997; Dinges et al. 1987; Dhand and Sohal 2006). But short naps (thirty to ninety minutes), particularly when taken around midday, increase functioning and help stave off low mood and cognitive problems (Kennedy et al. 2007; Monk et al. 2001; Takahashi, Fukuda, and Arito 1998). So proper napping turns out to be very helpful.

Now we'll move on to the next most common thing most of us do in bed (or used to, before we were parents). Let's take a look at sex.

Why We Have Sex, Why We Don't

Read any of the popular blogs about parenthood and one of the first things you'll find is some wistfulness about sex. They can sound a bit like, "Hey, remember when?" Not to scare you or anything, but the reality is that sex changes after a baby and will never be the same. It will be better in some ways, more familiar than when the relationship began, but still never the same.

Andi and Jaime were together for five years before they married, and they were married for almost eight before their first child was born. They were a fun couple, and their sex life was very satisfactory. Nothing you'd see in the DVDs from the back room of your local video store, mind you, but deeply satisfying and varied enough nonetheless. Sex was where they felt most connected and where they repaired their breaches.

When they became parents, Andi never could quite put her finger on when things shifted. Was it after their daughter's birth or sometime later, after their son joined the family? At first she tried initiating sex, but getting the brush-off from Jaime wore on her after a while. Andi backed off and waited to see how long it would take him to notice. Sadly, he never did. Or worse, he seemed relieved. Meanwhile, Jaime was busy with work. Once the babies started coming, his anxiety climbed. Jaime was determined to be a good father and, whether rational or not, he felt the burden of providing. And the more he pushed himself into the provider role, relegating the domestic domain to Andi, the more she resented the game switch. However much he achieved, Jaime was always straining for more. But more what? More security, more margin to buffer life's uncertainties, he supposed. In the old days, when it was just him and Andi, Jaime had been easygoing, always looking ahead to the next great vacation. Now, uncertainty dogged him. "What if" questions woke with him in the morning and spoke to him from the backseat on his drive home from work. The only real comfort he felt was at work, when he lost himself in the adrenaline haze of questions, demands, and deadlines that came lobbing at him in a steady, mind-numbing stream. Sitting still, turning his focus to his body, felt intrusive and irritating.

As Jaime grew more distant from his feelings and his body, sex slipped on his priority list and became more difficult for him. At first, if Andi worked on him long enough he could get there, but the effort seemed less and less worth the payoff. So, when Andi stopped asking, Jaime convinced himself that motherhood had changed Andi. What are the words of the poet? Ah yes, Sir Walter Scott: "Oh! what a tangled web we weave /When first we practice to deceive!" (*Marmion*, canto six, stanza 17, Sir Walter Scott). And of course, we usually deceive self first. By the time they came to see me in desperation over the state of their marriage, neither Jaime nor Andi could remember the last time they had made love.

As with sleep, it's important to consider what is normal for postpartum sexuality in order to understand its disruption. Of course, what is considered normal varies, but there are some trends that affect just about everyone with an infant at home. And the trend shouldn't surprise anyone—along with sleep deprivation comes a drop in sexual activity. Before we delve into the specifics of how sleep deprivation, diminished sexual contact, and depression intertwine after the stork, perhaps it could be helpful to consider the broader question. Why do we have sex?

The polite answer in our society is understood to be some variant of "because we love each other and it's fun." But would it surprise you to know that when researchers asked this question to basically random people, 203 men and 241 women ranging in age from seventeen to fifty-two, they got a total of 237 different and distinct reasons why people have sex? Of these 237 different reasons, 142 reasons were clearly represented by four broad factors and thirteen subfactors (Meston and Buss 2007). And would it surprise you to know that, for the most part, women have sex for the same reasons men do? It came as a surprise the writers at *Salon.com* (Clark-Flory 2009). Of course, there were also the expected differences in terms of the frequency each gender endorsed certain factors over others. So, men more often endorsed reasons having to do with physical appearance or wanting a new experience, and women more often endorsed reasons having to do with emotional closeness and commitment. These differences hold up the usual evolutionary arguments, or at least the deep cultural understanding that such arguments are true. But overall, both men and women like to have sex for many, many reasons, and chief among them is the desire for intimacy and closeness (Meston and Buss 2007).

In a way, the arrival of a baby focuses a couple's intimacy on this one compelling desire—the desire for closeness. But the exhaustion that characterizes the first several weeks—sometimes months—of parenthood (regardless of how baby comes into a family) shifts a couple's priorities away from genital expressions of intimacy toward emotional ones. This is true for biological and adoptive parents, couples gay and straight the world over (Gianino 2008; Ahlborg, Dahlof, and Hallberg 2005). Predictably, respondents noted a marked decline in sexual activity due either to exhaustion or to children sharing a bedroom with them, or both. "What was emphasized by some informants was that while sex had fallen off the radar, they simultaneously experienced enhanced feelings of intimacy" (Gianino 2008, 219). Indeed, when a couple can make this shift to sensuality and affection, sexuality is preserved and more easily reinstated later on. Sadly, as with Jaime and Andi, the disruptions in a couple's sexuality that begin after a baby's arrival can sometimes linger and deepen if the couple fails to redefine normal in a satisfactory way, a way that retains vibrancy and connection.

Let's explore how things work, how they can go wrong, and how you can minimize the problems and maximize the pleasure. How does desire work? What are the effects of pregnancy, anxiety, and body-image issues on sexuality?

Bridges to Desire

Clinical sex therapists have long known what empirical research is just beginning to show: that there are several bridges to sexual desire and both men and women are capable of accessing sexuality along multiple venues. True, men and women typically have different emphases, and female sexuality is apparently more flexible and responsive, but both men and women can access sexuality several different ways (McCarthy and McCarthy 2003; Baumeister 2000). These bridges include visual stimulation, emotional closeness, sensate focus, and erotic imagination. Keeping all four paths to desire and arousal open and functioning and adjusting expectations away from Hollywood models of fantastic sex to more realistic ones of good-enough sex can help a couple protect their sexuality from life's ups and downs (McCarthy and Thestrup 2009).

To complicate matters, when one partner is depressed (or when both are), sex can take even longer to get back online. Depression interferes with sexual desire, and antidepressants often interfere with sexual functioning (sometimes both arousal and orgasm but most commonly orgasm) (Frohlich and Meston 2005; DiScalea, Hanusa, and Wisner 2009; Ahrold and Meston 2009). Although the research literature that I could find studied only women's (lack of) sexual desire postpartum, in my clinical practice I have seen new dads with low desire or other sexual difficulties like erectile failure and premature or delayed ejaculation that began after the baby arrived. The effect of anxiety, stress hormones, and couvade on male sexual functioning apparently hasn't caught the attention of the scientific research community just yet.

Desire and the Physicality of Birth and Mothering

All of that research on postpartum sexuality focusing on women explores the effects of breastfeeding on sexual desire and when the average couple resumes sexual relations after pregnancy. Indeed, the hormonal changes involved in breastfeeding (lower testosterone and androstenedione) plays some role in women's sexual desire and sexual functioning (Abdool, Thakar, and Sultan 2009). Women who breastfeed also report that getting less sleep, having sore nipples, and feeling a sense of "touch overload" all influence their lack of sexual desire (Ahlborg, Dahlof, and Hallberg 2005). In general, breastfeeding women tend to have less interest in sex relative to bottle-feeding mothers, and this usually lasts for the duration of nursing (Alder 1989; Abdool, Thakar, and Sultan 2009). But there are significant differences found across cultures. So, while 53 percent of British women report lower sexual desire three months postpartum, 62 percent of Nigerian women do (Abdool, Thakar, and Sultan 2009). I couldn't find any statistics on Hispanic women, but given the extraordinarily low rates of postpartum depression among Latinas it seems likely that cultural differences might be even more apparent if we had information about postpartum sexual desire in this and other groups (Wei et al. 2008). After all, beliefs and expectancies are tremendously important in shaping expressions of sexuality, and culture forms most of our beliefs and expectancies. So, logically, we would expect culture to play a significant role in shaping sexual behaviors, including when a couple resumes sexual intimacy after a baby. However, we don't have much cross-cultural data on this.

Giving birth is a major physical feat, no matter how many (cruel) stories we've all heard about women who give birth in the morning and are back plowing in the afternoon. Biological mothers typically need a period of time to heal physically before resuming sexual activity, whether the birth was vaginal and without perineal tearing, vaginal with tearing or with episiotomy, or by C-section. Women who give birth resume sexual intercourse, on average, by about six to seven weeks postpartum (Alder 1989). The majority (88 percent) have resumed intercourse by twelve weeks. Interestingly, on average, sexual contact that does not involve intercourse occurs within two or three weeks after the birth (1989). Overall, sexual desire and frequency of intercourse are typically back to prepregnancy or pre-baby levels by one year postpartum (Barrett et al. 2000; Signorello et al. 2001; VonSydow 1999).

Anxiety and Sex

Some people seem to find a little anxiety stimulating; other people find that even a little anxiety shuts down the sexual response cycle. This apparent contradiction has baffled sexologists for decades (Hoon, Wincze, and Hoon 1977). But when researchers started distinguishing between *state anxiety* (momentary, situational anxiety), *trait anxiety* (what you might call being "high strung"), and *sensitivity to anxiety* (fear of anxiety itself), the picture began to come into focus. These three dimensions of anxiety turn out to be very different and to have very different effects on sexual responses (Bradford and Meston 2006; Palace and Gorzalka 1990). Human sexuality is very complex and very heavily influenced by mental and attitudinal factors (VonSydow 2002; Basson 2002b, 2003; Basson et al. 2003). Women who are high-strung, temperamentally prone to anxiety, "reported less frequent, consistent, and/or satisfying mental sexual arousal ('turn on') during sexual activity but no impairment in vaginal lubrication," suggesting that anxious women experience sexual difficulties even though they get aroused physically—their anxiety distracts them from their own pleasure (Bradford and Meston 2006). In contrast, women who are not so predisposed to be anxious, who are more laid-back, are the ones who benefit from the enhancing effects of a *moderate situational anxiety*, meaning the kind of emotional tension, the sympathetic nervous system (SNS) arousal, that makes "doing it" in the backseat of a car exciting for some. This is the kind of arousal that makes grabbing a quickie while the kids are napping exciting to some. And it's also the kind of arousal that you might experience after intense exercise (Bradford and Meston 2006). We don't yet have similar studies or data on the effect of anxiety on men.

Body Image and Sexuality

Performance anxiety affects male sexuality, often producing erectile difficulties, premature ejaculation, or inhibited ejaculation. Body image matters a great deal to women (Seal and Meston 2007; Pauls, Occhino, and Dryfhout 2008; Pauls et al. 2008). In fact, some sexologists believe that body-image disturbance in women is roughly analogous to performance anxiety in men—both result in disruption of the sexual-response cycle (Seal and Meston 2007). To top it all off, if sleep deprivation is prolonged and sleep quality poor, if sleep deprivation is compounded by depression, metabolic changes can occur that make losing baby weight—those added pounds from pregnancy—difficult (Spiegel et al. 2009; Leproult and Van Cauter 2010). And persistent pounds have a tremendous impact on body image (Boyington, Johnson, and Carter-Edwards 2007; Clark et al. 2009; Shrewsbury et al. 2009). Of course pregnancy changes a woman's body, and delivery in particular can shift her anatomy in key ways. But the impact of such changes on body image and on postpartum sexuality has only recently become a focus of serious scientific inquiry (Rallis et al. 2007). On average, half of the women who were surveyed about their sexual adjustment after delivery reported body-image problems (Pastore, Owens, and Raymond 2007). African-American women had better body imagery than did Caucasian women, as is true generally (Pauls et al. 2008; Boyington, Johnson, and Carter-Edwards 2007). Interestingly, these problems persisted well into the postpartum period, long after the women had returned to their prepregnancy weight and had healed from any physical trauma of labor and delivery (Pauls et al. 2008). And while self-objectification and body imagery have been studied in men, I don't know of any studies asking heterosexual men about the effect of couvade weight gain on their body image and sexuality after a baby, or on a man's difficulties losing weight due to sleep deprivation and/ or depression postnatally (Hargreaves and Tiggemann 2009; Galli and Reel 2009; Kozak, Frankenhauser, and Roberts 2009).

Based on my clinical work, I have some ideas about what some of these changes might mean and why they persist, though of course these thoughts require further research. First, I suspect that some women disconnect from their bodies during pregnancy or as a result of difficult labor much the same way that trauma survivors and people who undergo lengthy or painful medical treatments disconnect from their physicality (Brotto, Basson, and Luria 2008; Haven and Pearlman 2004). It's entirely possible that some men might respond this way to witnessing their wives give birth, but we don't know. And sleep deprivation also comes into play in several ways. Disruptions in certain kinds of brain functions during sleep likely interfere with cognitive and emotional flexibility, the flexibility necessary to fully embrace changes in body imagery (Leproult and Van Cauter 2010; Walker 2009). Fortunately, treatment approaches that aim to increase body awareness and acceptance are highly successful (Cash, Maikkula, and Yamamiya 2004; Cash 1997).

The Sexy Brain

In one recent study, female volunteers viewing an erotic film had higher levels of sexual arousal if experimenters had instructed them to imagine they had positive feelings about sexuality and about their own sexual responsiveness (these are known as *positive sexual schemas*). Even volunteers who were depressed, as measured by various pre-tests, responded positively (Kuffel and Heiman 2006). These authors concluded that it is useful to know that the effects of your thoughts on sexual arousal can be quite immediate (Kuffel and Heiman 2006). They then did the study again, this time using volunteers who were not depressed but who did have a formal diagnosis of female sexual arousal disorder (FSAD). These women enjoyed the same results—adopting a positive schema for the purposes of the experiment, *imagining* they had positive attitudes about sex in general and their own sexuality in particular, made a big difference in both their subjective and objective levels of arousal (Middleton, Kuffel, and Heiman 2008). In fact, the only real difference between the "normal" group (volunteers who did not have any sexual problems) and the FSAD group were their attitudes toward sex and sexuality: Women with FSAD perceived their sexuality significantly more negatively than sexually healthy women (Middleton, Kuffel, and Heiman 2008).

This research supports a current understanding of sexual arousal as information processing. The idea is that sexual arousal begins with some relevant information (a lover's flirtatious remarks, a caress— that kind of thing) that the brain then sorts in memory. When the information links up with sexual meaning in the brain, automatic processes activate genital responses. But when the information also accesses nonsexual memories and/or negative meanings, then sexual arousal may be low and negative and emotions might interfere (Kuffel and Heiman 2006). Again, we don't know how much this applies to male sexuality because the researchers haven't studied that yet. But the importance, one might even say primacy, of attitude over physiology, at least in female sexuality, is further highlighted by studies on the effects of anxiety on female sexual arousal and by pharmacological studies in search of drugs that might be the counterpart for Viagra in women.

What You Can Do

If you are a man and you experience erectile difficulties, a PDE-5 inhibitor such as Viagra, Levitra, or Cialis can help (and many urologists privately believe that the placebo effect is powerful with these drugs). If you are a man and experience premature ejaculation, an SSRI can help. Although it is considered an "off label" use of these drugs, physicians often prescribe SSRIs to men with PE because one of the most reliable side effects is to disrupt or delay the ability to climax (Ahrold and Meston 2009). But the search for a pharmacological key to female desire shows just how little women's sexuality really has to do with genital blood flow or mere physiology (Bradford and Meston 2009). Wellbutrin was originally thought to be the goose with the golden egg, but it turned out to be better used as an antidepressant instead. Wellbutrin is helpful for quitting smoking and is often prescribed as an antidepressant when the physician wants to avoid the negative sexual side effects common to SSRIs, but it's ineffective in producing sexual desire or arousal (Ahrold and Meston 2009). Viagra also had a go as an off-label treatment for women's sexual arousal and desire problems—for a short while. "Although laboratory studies indicate that, for the most part, these drugs performed as expected physiologically by facilitating genital vasocongestive responses [directing bloodflow to the genital area], in most studies they did not affect a comparable increase in psychological sexual arousal (Bradford and Meston 2009, 165).

Freud never did figure out the answer to the question about what women want, and so far Big Pharma isn't doing much better. The drugs work—they have the intended physiological effect; but they don't work—they don't change subjective, emotional arousal any better than placebo (Bradford and Meston 2009). This suggests that, once again, expectancy effects rule—that is, the women in these studies reacted because they believe pills work and expected that these pills would do the trick. The placebo effect happens because we pay closer attention to our body's natural fluctuations and magnify whatever little evidence we find that supports our hope, our desire, our expectancy that "by golly, it's working!"

Female desire, in all its mystery, is governed and influenced by a myriad of factors. Early sex researchers Masters and Johnson believed that desire always precedes arousal, and this is usually true—for men.

But newer research shows that this model is not so true for women. Women often experience desire *after* arousal begins (Basson 2002a; Brotto, Basson, and Woo 2009; Basson 2001). This model gives a much larger role to mental factors and thus expands the possibilities for treatment of interrupted desire (Kuffel and Heiman 2006; Middleton, Kuffel, and Heiman 2008). So, for postpartum couples it may be helpful to schedule sexual encounters, to plan for them, to flirt, anticipate, and fantasize about them in order to encourage desire and protect the couple's sexual connection.

Visual stimulation is salient to both men and women, but male sexuality tends to be more dependent on the visual channel (Baumeister 2000). The emotional channel is also available to both men and women, but women's sexuality tends to depend on emotional closeness to a greater degree than does male sexuality (McCarthy and McCarthy 2003; Andersen, Cyranowski, and Aarestad 2000). *Sensate focus* is a fancy term for an intense attention to sensuality and touch, sometimes supplemented with erotic imagination or fantasy, and couples can use this emphasis to cultivate a sense of playfulness in the bedroom (LoPiccolo and LoPiccolo 1978; LoPiccolo and Stock 1986; Perel 2007).

Depression, anxiety, sleep disturbance, and disruptions of sexual functioning are all intricately, elegantly, and mysteriously interconnected. Stresses that hit one area spill over into another. Solutions to one can compound another, which is why it is so very important to take all the myriad interwoven threads into consideration in treatment and why simple solutions usually don't last long. This complexity is also why psychologists train for eight or more years and need many more years of clinical experience before achieving proficiency in the artistry of therapy.

Yet couples often don't appear on the radar of medical professionals, in part because they don't complain to their doctor or seek out a sex therapist right away. Most of the couples I see in my practice have been struggling, crawling on their bellies over broken glass, trying to solve the problem on their own for years before they ever think to seek treatment, and then only because divorce looms large on the horizon. Seeing these efforts in my practice, I'm both awed by the tenacity of the human spirit and saddened about the years of joy, vibrancy, and connection so often lost to unnecessary suffering.

Let's revisit Andi and Jaime to see what steps they took to solve their problem. Once they had faced the fact that they needed help and came to me, Andi and Jaime began by protecting their at-home conversations—saving the uncomfortable talk about problems that needed to be solved for specific, pre-appointed times and taking care to keep their attitude, outlook, and words positive otherwise. Jaime began to look for ways to participate in home care and parenting instead of waiting for Andi to ask and ask again, as if the home was her domain. Andi took care to notice Jaime's efforts and to thank him; Jaime did the same. They made deliberate efforts to reconnect with family and friends, broadening their circle and intentionally cultivating social ties. Eventually they found ways to trade babysitting with other parents so that they could make date night a regular occurrence. They woke up a little earlier in the morning so they could have their coffee together in the den before the kids woke up. They set aside time to hold each other naked, in a full frontal embrace for ten to fifteen minutes before getting dressed and getting off to work, and then pondered the touch, the smell, the laughter of the morning at random intervals during the day. They scheduled their sexual encounters and planned for them, letting go of the romantic illusion of spontaneous combustion *and* the resentment that life had to be a little more structured for now. They each looked for ways to show affection and stopped expecting sex to always involve intercourse and orgasm. Andi was surprised at how much more relaxed she felt and how much easier the kids seemed to be. Jaime rediscovered just how much he enjoyed his body and took up running again. He even found reasons to leave work at work and come down off his adrenaline high. Once they were getting along better, once they each felt loved and held again, they began to talk. Andi and Jaime started talking, really talking well, before they started having intercourse again.

Change didn't come in a bottle and it didn't happen overnight, but together Andi and Jaime began to shape a vision for how life could be full, rich, and rewarding and how they could buffer the strains of life—what we call stress—by building a satisfying family life grounded in the intimacy of their marriage.

Even though you, like Andi and Jaime, are likely to find sleep and sex to be different after the stork, unlike Andi and Jaime, you don't have to let the drift set in before you take steps to heal it. You can actively work to prepare yourself for the changes to come and take steps to keep the fun and sensuality alive in your relationship. You can practice good sleep hygiene and train yourself to become a better sleeper. You can protect your conversation and schedule your problem-solving talks. You can make a point of being thoughtful and playful, and you can cultivate erotic imagination well before or even after the baby joins the family. The exercises at the end of this chapter are designed to help you do these things.

Exercises for Chapter 5

Basic Principles of Sleep Hygiene

As you now know, setting up strategies and rituals to help you get to sleep (and stay asleep) is a great way for you to address your sleep issues. Consider the points of sleep hygiene, below, and work to implement them into your life.

- The bed is only for two things—sleeping and making love. Keep the TV out of the bedroom.

- Do not read in bed—ever.

- Exercise in the middle of the day, not at the end. Nap in the morning or early afternoon, not later.

- Stay away from stimulants: TV, alcohol, caffeine, arguments, and intense emotions, especially late in the day.

- If sleep eludes you for ten minutes, get out of bed and go into another room. Meditation is better than rumination and approximates the benefits of sleep in terms of brain waves, so try some meditating while on hiatus from your bed.

Exercise 1:
Develop a Bedtime Routine

Begin the day with curiosity (in order to prime your unconscious mind to notice positive things) and end the day with gratitude: Review the small victories, accomplishments, and pleasant events. Find the silver lining in any negative events that might have occurred.

While lying in your bed waiting for sleep to come, practice mindfulness, body awareness, or other relaxation exercises. Learn a poem or prayer by heart, then repeat it to yourself instead of ruminating. Schedule a time to worry, then put off worrying until your scheduled worry time.

If you can't get to sleep within ten minutes, get out of bed and go to another room. While there, listen to soothing music, drink hot herbal tea, hot milk, or hot water with honey and lemon juice, and try meditating. But stay in the dark, keeping your mind empty, until you are ready to return to bed to fall asleep. Some studies suggest that insomniacs might actually get a little sleep but not be aware of it—their self-report is at odds with the physiological measures (Nelson and Harvey 2003).

Listen to a tape or CD of hypnosis for sleep.

Exercise 2: Strategies for
Stopping Rumination

If you are a ruminator, you'll need to develop several strategies to help you break the pattern once it starts. With practice you will be able to turn out of the tailspin that is rumination more and more quickly.

Visualize a stop sign in your mind and hear yourself saying "stop that" very sharply and authoritatively. Wear a rubber band on your wrist and snap it against your wrist if necessary to make the association—rumination hurts your brain, so stop it!

Train yourself to sing "Stop in the Name of Love" *out loud* every time the cascade of ruminations starts. This strategy works best if you have a terrible voice and are embarrassed to sing in public, but it can be helpful even if you happen to be the next Norah Jones or Josh Groban. And if you're just not going to sing out loud, or you're in a crowded elevator somewhere, humming will work too.

Visualize an emotionally neutral scene in your mind. Now visualize that same scene as if it's on a television screen. Now find a little button in the lower right-hand corner of the screen, then turn the button until the screen shrinks. Keep shrinking the screen until it is very tiny. Now turn it off. Repeat this as many times as you need to until you can get your hands on the control buttons quickly and easily.

The next time you catch yourself making up a fantastical story in your mind about all the bad things that could happen to your baby, stop, turn off the negative imagery, and change the channel in your mind. Now begin to make up a fantastically *positive* story about all the wonderful things that could happen to your baby. Notice that both stories are imaginary and that *you* control your imagination. Since you're in control, you can choose to make up great stories or lousy ones, but neither one is reality. Thoughts are just thoughts.

The next time you catch yourself asking "what if ..." followed by some terrible scenario, answer the question. Make a rule and follow it: You only get to ask "what if" questions if you are going to answer the question. Hint: If something terrible happens, then you will feel awful. And you'll get over it. Such is life. Also remember that worrying actually doesn't stop bad things from happening, nor does it save you from dealing with bad feelings afterward if they do happen.

Set aside a time to worry. Make it a very specific time and limit the time frame to just a few minutes; ten minutes should be sufficient. Any worries that come up at any other time must wait until the next day's worry time. So, if you decide that your worry time is every morning from 6:00 to 6:10 a.m., when a worry pops up at three o'clock in the afternoon, you have to tell yourself to hold that thought until tomorrow at worry time.

Exercise 4:
Sensuality and Playfulness

Here are some tips and strategies to help you enrich your sensual and sexual connection with your partner. Some of them may feel odd or even a little uncomfortable at first, but make a decision to give each one a try. Once you get over the initial unfamiliarity, I'm guessing you'll begin to enjoy this time.

Couch Time

Set aside some time to sit on the sofa or somewhere else comfortable with your honey. Gaze into each other's eyes without speaking. Synchronize your breathing. Now switch up who leads and who follows with the breath. Try to do this without giggling, but don't worry if you occasionally erupt—you'll get better with practice.

Un-Sex Safe Time

Set aside some time to embrace one another in a full frontal embrace—naked. This is protected time, which means that no matter what comes up, you vow intercourse will not happen. Developing anticipation and letting sexual tension build gently and gradually is important to cultivating intimacy and enhancing blood flow to the genitals, but it also helps to expand your sensual and sexual awareness so that your genitals can be more sensitive when you do decide to resume.

Planned Sex

Plan your sexual encounters, schedule them, and make them a priority. Drop the baby off with your best friend, mother, sister, aunt Eunice, or favorite MMO (mother's morning out) location. Change the sheets, light mildly scented candles, take a shower or bath together before or after. Focus on all five senses and take your time to really let your touch communicate love. Studies show that people can actually identify emotions quite reliably just through the sense of touch (Hertenstein et al. 2009). When your touch is saying "love," you're not only providing safety and comfort, you're actually catching it—love is contagious too.

CHAPTER 6

The Dance of Parenting

There isn't any formula or method. You learn to love by loving.

Aldous Huxley

Several years ago, Stephen Covey sparked a movement in time management and personal goal setting. His book *The Seven Habits of Highly Effective People* has sold over fifteen million copies and has been translated into thirty-eight different languages. The second principle that he identifies is the principle of personal vision; in other words, to "begin with the end in mind" (Covey 1989, 13). But what does it mean to begin with the end in mind when it comes to raising babies?

The goal of parenting is to raise children who will become independent adults, who will go on to love, to work, and to contribute to society. It will be years before you see evidence of character in your little one and decades before you know whether she is successful (whatever that means). And, of course, standards for success are culturally constructed and change over time. In Colonial America the standards of success were different than they were in Victorian times. During the Great Depression success for many was redefined in terms of mere survival. Since the 1950s, success in our culture has increasingly been constructed in material terms of wealth and education. The skills necessary to survive a covered-wagon journey from the eastern seaboard to the great, untamed west were arguably different from the skills necessary to navigate multicultural complexities in a global economy connected by computers and the Internet. Or are they?

Parenting: The Ambiguities

We all want what's best for our children. This is not new, not a particular value of the modern world we now inhabit. What *is* new, what *is* particular to this time in history is just how ambiguous the standard is (Costner 1960). Go to Amazon.com and type in a search for books on "parenting" and you'll get more than a hundred thousand results. And that's just what's available on one popular bookseller's website! Americans are bombarded with books on parenting but, as a very heterogeneous culture, we lack the kind of clear, coherent mores typical of other, more traditional societies (or even America in past periods). The global village is filled with contradictions, and there are no reliable signposts on the information highway.

How should we evaluate such a plethora of information? It can be comforting to imagine that all these different opinions have equal merit, but do they? We might borrow parenting strategies out of context from other cultures, hoping that our parenting practices will result in happy, successful children, children who embody our currently popular character values of confidence and good self-esteem. But hope is not a strategy. I'd like to make the case that, across cultures and throughout history, one skill set is fundamental—the skills necessary to regulate one's own emotional experience. The ability to regulate one's behaviors naturally flows out of the skills enabling emotion regulation. And once a child can regulate his emotions and behaviors, he's prepared for success in getting along with others, mastering the tools of the culture, and negotiating the rules of the society in which he lives.

As you consider all the choices that face you and will face you in the future as a parent, as you consider your value system and your best wishes for your little one, it could be easy to get overwhelmed. But I'd like for you to consider this: whatever wonderful things you wish for the future of this baby, they are mostly outside of your control. The one thing that you *can* shape is how well this baby learns to regulate her own emotional experience. If you take this goal to heart as your basic framework, I believe that the overwhelming array of choices and ambiguities will become more manageable. Everything I have to say about parenting is ultimately geared toward helping you sort through the many contradictory cultural messages, choices, and expectations that you will face with one goal in mind: teaching your child how to regulate his own emotional experience.

Everything else—whether she will like school or he will enjoy sports, whether she is mechanically inclined or he has an artist's eye, how much education he will grow up to attain or how much money she will earn—are not your cards to play. Whether you enroll her in Suzuki or Montessori, whether he has a nanny who speaks Chinese or Spanish or both, there are still no guarantees. Welcome to parenthood. The bad news is that parenthood is a minefield of ambiguities; the good news is that it is *not all up to you*. An old Arab proverb says "men resemble the times more than they resemble their fathers," and that, alas, is true (Twenge 2006, 3). You have an important charge, and your influence is important—but it isn't everything. Many, many variables will impact your child during his lifetime. So, if one way to reduce ambiguity is to clarify goals and expectations, perhaps we should begin by defining some reasonable goals. If we can agree on the first goal of imparting skills for self-regulation, then we can begin to talk about how to do this. Instead of offering specifics, I would like to simply offer a fundamental principle: the principle of attunement.

Attunement

Attunement is a very broad concept that refers to how responsive you and your baby are to one another's cues. Attunement is a very subtle quality of emotional connection between caregiver and infant. The very basis of the parent–child bond is their attunement, and the quality of this attunement will set the tone for the relationship for years to come. This dynamic is sometimes called *synchrony*, and it has biological aspects that begin in utero, when a mother and her baby's biorhythms accommodate to one another (Feldman 2006, 186). Synchrony is defined as "an ongoing match in the mother's and infant's direction of involvement in the interaction" and is likened to a dance (Feldman 2006, 177).

Sophisticated technology now exists that permits developmental neuroscientists to measure minute time lags in the exchange of social and emotional cues between mom and baby, cues involving eye contact, smiling, and even heartbeat (Feldman 2006). Researchers first videotape the parent–child interactions and observe them in slow-motion playback. The researchers break the tapes into three-second segments, coding the details of the interaction with great precision. Using these micro-synchrony measures, researchers are able to determine who is "driving" the interaction—leading the dance, as it were. In highly synchronous pairs, baby initiates many of these interactions by three months, indicating that the caregiver is "responsive to microlevel shifts in the infant's affective state" (Feldman 2006, 178). These highly sophisticated measures of micro-level synchrony show disruption in parent–infant pairs when the parent is depressed or when the infant was born very prematurely (Field et al. 1990; Feldman 2006). By comparing the development of various biological rhythms (or *oscillators*) in premature babies to full-term infants, researchers are able to determine that the baby doesn't simply respond to the mother's lead in developing synchrony. Rather, "the organization of biological rhythms, the infant's capacity to orient to the environment, and the ability to regulate arousal efficiently all contribute meaningfully to the formation of mother-infant second-by-second synchrony" (Feldman 2006, 184). And although maternal–infant synchrony is disturbed both when the caretaker is depressed and when the baby is premature, these difficulties are repairable. In fact, "when the mothers were no longer depressed at the six-month interaction period, the infants were also no longer depressed" (Field et al. 1990, 13). And the preemies were back on par with their full-term peers at age-adjusted 3 months when they had a mother who "led" the dance with sensitivity. This result prompted the author of the study to conclude "that with development, biology and context shape each other in a mutually influencing manner, and more favorable environments may function to attenuate the effects of major physiological delays" (Feldman 2006).

Cultivating Attunement

Since you don't have the fancy equipment at home to measure micro-level synchrony between you and your baby, what you get to do instead is *notice*. Noticing the subtle nuances in your baby's cues and seeing how well your baby notices your cues is the next level of attunement. When you make eye contact with the baby, do you smile? Can you distinguish between a tired cry and a hungry cry? When your attunement with your baby is stronger, you'll be able to accurately distinguish between different facial expressions, cries, and other behaviors. And as you begin to recognize which behavior means what, you'll feel more confident in your decisions—you will have the categories and criteria you need to keep your own anxieties at bay. So, for instance, you'll be able to avoid confusing the baby by feeding her when she's tired. Or, you'll be comfortable allowing her to cry a little while when she's gotten overstimulated and needs to discharge tension so she can get to sleep.

Being able to distinguish between different cries is an important example because it demonstrates how a strong attunement with your baby—including being able to categorize her behaviors accurately—will help you determine what she truly needs. A strong attunement will allow you to know with confidence when your crying baby needs feeding, or needs soothing, or whether it's time to allow her to struggle a bit in order to learn to soothe herself to sleep.

It is through attunement that the parent knows just what little bit of struggle is enough and when it becomes too much. Attunement is the means by which you find the balance point. If you ever learned to drive a stick shift, you know what it is to search for the sweet spot where you let your foot off the clutch just enough to shift gears. If you've ever learned to dance a partner dance, then you know what it is to feel where your balance point is, where your partner is in relation to your lead, or, if you are a follower, where your partner is leading. These things cannot be learned from reading a book or even from observing others do the behavior. Learning these things requires a different kind of attention, tuning into cues from your body and emotions in addition to purely visual evidence. And these kinds of learning require coordination of internal cues (your own kinesthetic information) with external data (visual and auditory input about things outside of yourself). In the case of standard driving, you must learn to feel where the balance point is and coordinate that internal information with external visual and auditory cues to engage the gear and move through traffic. In the case of dancing, you must learn to attend to your own sensory and physical cues and coordinate them with visual, auditory, and tactile cues about your partner, the music, and others on the dance floor. When it comes to parenting, you learn to attend to your own emotional state and to a wide range of information, including the baby's emotional cues and information that you pick up through all available senses. Attunement later becomes the foundation for "other-person" perspective taking, the capacity to understand the child's behavior from the child's point of view.

Attachment Theory

Attunement is the basis for what we have come to know as "attachment styles," and the concept of attachment styles comes from attachment theory. This theory, as set forth by researchers John Bowlby and Mary Ainsworth, is hugely important in the history of psychology and the understanding of human development.

In the modern age, there have been many ideas and theories about how children develop and how best to raise them. For instance, before attachment theory there was psychoanalytic theory. Child analysts like Melanie Klein taught that the emotional problems of young children stemmed from internal conflicts between aggressive and libidinal urges rather than from problems in the environment or family relationships (Bretherton 1992).

John Bowlby, a psychoanalytically trained psychiatrist, was interested in the impact of maternal separation on personality development. Mary Ainsworth, a psychologist, did her dissertation on personality dimensions of security and independence as they related to mature or immature defenses. Later in her career she developed the "stranger situation," an experimental method for assessing how securely infants were attached to their caregivers based on how much anxiety they showed when exposed to a stranger or to mother's absence. Ainsworth identified several patterns thought to reflect the degree of confidence and security the infant feels toward the caregiver. These patterns have come to be known as *attachment styles.*

Ainsworth noticed that the infants who appeared most securely attached cried very little when they were introduced to strangers or exposed to novel stimuli, and they were easy to distract and soothe when their mother was absent for brief periods of time. She also noticed that these same infants had mothers who were very sensitive to the infant's cues (Bretherton 1992; Ainsworth 1979; Ainsworth and Bowlby 1991).

This notion of attunement is the key point of attachment theory. But pop culture takes attachment theory out of context and distorts it into prescriptions for breastfeeding, mother-only care, and co-sleeping—prescriptions that are way out of line with the original research. Mary Ainsworth herself, perhaps sensing the potential for her work to be distorted and misrepresented, wrote in 1979 "[d]espite a steady increase in our understanding of the complexities of response to and effects of separation from attachment figures in infancy and early childhood, it is difficult to suggest clear-cut guidelines for parents and others responsible for infant and child care." She went on to specifically state "[m]any have interpreted Bowlby's attachment theory as claiming that an infant can become attached to only one person—the mother. This is a mistaken interpretation" (Ainsworth 1979, 935).

How Important Are Early Influences?

You may take some hope from the knowledge that, no matter which parenting strategy you choose, it alone cannot and will not determine adult personality development. In other words, whether you co-sleep or don't, whether you breastfeed for two full years or not, none of these strategies will determine your child's ultimate personality. Research shows that personality continues to change until about age thirty (some say fifty), after which it is mostly (but not entirely) stable. So, you won't be "ruining" your child forever if you choose the "wrong" strategy. You also won't be guaranteeing your child a marvelous personality if you choose the "right" strategy. No matter what you do, your child's personality will continue to develop throughout his life and into adulthood. Long-range, aggregate studies of the personality stability literature suggest a stability rate of about 75 percent (Ferguson 2010). "Overall, corrected stability coefficients suggested that the stability of personality across adulthood is high, with only modest change. By contrast, personality during childhood is significantly more changeable" (Ferguson 2010, 659) And a really interesting twist is that the apparent stability of the adult personality may largely be a function of the fact that adults are more likely to have choices about their environment and to choose environments that suit (and maintain) their personality structure (Bandura 2006). Also interesting is that these statistics hold for many Western cultures (American, Canadian, and European) but not all. The stability coefficients for people in the South Pacific are lower, suggesting that culture and expectancies can also play a role.

But early influences have long been overstated in the popular imagination. A pamphlet written in 1851 claimed, "By the mother's forming hand the child receives its shape to a great extent for all its future existence" (Kagan 1996, 901). So, while attunement and attachment are important, the fact remains that human beings are remarkably resilient. Children who grew up in horrific circumstances such as Nazi concentration camps and Bengali slums not only have survived but have also gone on to thrive as productive citizens. Pop culture today over-reaches the research data on attachment, despite many decades of hard science, to carry on this centuries-old claim that early life experiences exert unchangeable influence in shaping human personality.

Jerome Kagan, one of the key pioneers of developmental psychology, holds an endowed chair and is professor emeritus at Harvard University. His research has helped us understand the stability of infant temperament over time and how infant temperament interacts with parenting styles. Kagan notes that the "pleasing idea" that "infants can create schemata, habits, and emotions that are enduring, perhaps indefinitely" has existed in one form or another for centuries. And although attachment is important, it is *not* at all warranted to suppose that early social experiences produce anything like unchangeable structures in the human brain. In fact, "[t]he evidence from many prospective longitudinal studies suggests that it is not until six or seven years of age that prediction of a large number of adult behaviors becomes substantial" (Kagan 1996, 902). It just doesn't fit with the empirical evidence we have about brain plasticity and human resiliency (Kagan 1996).

Choosing Strategies

Now that we're working with a clear goal (imparting skills for self-regulation) and a foundational principle (the principle of attunement), you'll have an easier time sorting through the parenting strategies available to you. You've also gained some perspective about how much control you actually have over how your child turns out. Now I'd like to provide some further perspective about how culture affects how we parent. By considering the cultural framework of our basic life decisions, we can see how relatively flexible our choices are. With no hard-and-fast rules (except, perhaps, to love your child), you can operate according to what works best for your family.

Cultural Context Matters

Historically and psychologically, parenting strategies grow out of a culture—parenting practices express the culture's deeply held core values and are, in turn, supported *by* the entirety of that culture. Consider two very traditional societies with very clear and very uniform practices for breastfeeding—the Dakota and the Yurok, as studied by Erik Erikson in the 1950s. The traditional custom of the Dakota held that infants and small children were to be nursed on demand for as long as they chose, usually from three to five years. In contrast, the Yurok were to wean at six or seven months, when the child begins to have teeth and is able to eat solid food. If we believe the myths (and the implications of the myths that parenting practices determine tribal or national character), we might expect that the Dakota became naturally peace loving because they were "secure," having been breastfed on demand. In reality, the Dakota were fierce warriors; the Yurok were conflict-avoidant fisherfolk (Erikson 1950). Of course, with the enormous changes these two cultures have undergone in the past sixty years, these characterizations may or may not still hold true.

However, these observations led Erikson to make two important points. The first is that child training strategies do *not* bear a direct, causal relationship to specific character traits. You cannot "format" your child's personality. Parenting strategies result in character traits like ferocity or conflict avoidance (or compassion) only because

175

multiple layers of *meaning* converge around the commonly held values that organize and define the culture. The second and most important point is that parenting strategies work when and if the parents communicate in *all* their actions that they really believe there is meaning to what they're doing. "Ultimately, children become neurotic not from frustrations, but from the lack or loss of societal meaning in these frustrations" (Erikson 1950, 249).

In order for the parents to communicate that they really believe there is meaning to what they are doing, they have to actually believe there *is* meaning to what they are doing, and that meaning has to extend beyond the couple, beyond the cult or the compound to the greater society. This is why the neither the Amish of Pennsylvania, nor the Mormons of Utah, nor the Davidians of Texas, nor any other group can really ever be entirely successful at imparting their values by isolating themselves. Children eventually encounter the larger world, and when they do, idiosyncratic and countercultural norms will not hold much sway.

The good news here is that there is a great deal of latitude in what works well. When you choose your parenting strategies, you get to consider what works for *you* as well as what works for the baby in the larger context of the culture in which you're parenting. Today's parents seem to experience a great deal of guilt over choosing what works best for them. But if you're not functioning well, you won't be the best parent you can be. Trying to squeeze yourself or your kid into some fad or formula is probably a good way to make yourself miserable, and in the long run, it's not likely to work very well for the baby either. For one thing, if your strategy doesn't fit you well, you're much more likely to wind up struggling with depression and shadowboxing with guilt for not doing what you think others think you should do.

The Target to Aim for: Firm but Yielding

In our culture, young children are expected to have basic skills for tolerating distress and self-soothing. By age five or six, most American children are expected to be autonomous enough to leave home and travel with other children, often on a bus, to attend a school. There they will sit still for long periods of time, listen to a teacher, answer when spoken to, participate in class, raise their hands to ask questions, and hold their own on the playground with physically active and some-times aggressive peers. These behavioral and interpersonal skills will necessitate a foundation in emotional self-regulation.

There is research to support the idea that a firm but yielding approach can help kids gain this kind of self-sufficiency at the relatively young age at which we expect it of them. Researcher Jerome Kagan looked at infants of different temperaments to see how this sort of approach worked. In his work, Kagan identified a continuum of infant temperament anchored on each extreme by characteristic responses to novel stimuli. The "high reactive" infants are those who respond to their environment with vigorous motor activity or vocalizing. About 20 percent of healthy newborns can be characterized as high reactives. The "low reactive" infants show very low levels of motor activity and minimal distress to the same events. About 40 percent of newborns can be characterized as low reactives.

Kagan found that the more highly reactive infants tend to become inhibited by two years of age, and the less reactive babies become sociable, less inhibited, and bolder by age two. These temperamental differences are rooted in biology and are largely inherited, having to do with the excitability of the amygdala and the amygdala's projections to other parts of the brain like the brain stem and the autonomic nervous system (Kagan 2000).

But it's important to remember that "although genes may make a modest contribution to these temperamental profiles, biology always shares power with experience" (Kagan 2000, 36). Within this study, an interesting interaction between infant temperament and parenting style occurs. The mothers of high reactive infants who were very *firm* and set *clear limits* helped their children overcome the tendency to be shy and fearful. Conversely, the mothers of highly reactive infants who were very gentle, yielding, and overly solicitous with their baby seemed to *exacerbate* the child's fears. By the time they were toddlers, the highly reactive infants raised with a permissive style were fearful, shy, and timid (Kagan, Arcus, and Snidman 1993; Kagan 1997, 2000).

Although the tools of the culture—reading, writing, and arith-metic—will, for most, be taught in school, the foundational skills of self-regulation will be learned at home. And training in the founda-tional skills of self-regulation will begin in infancy as interactions with caregivers begin to shape the baby's expectancies about feeding and sleep. This is why, given the demands and reward structure of our culture, it is sensible to aim for firm but attuned parenting.

Training Baby to Sleep

French babies sleep through the night sooner than do Italian babies (Romito, Sauren-Cubizolles, and Lelong 1999). Possibly because French parents *expect* the baby to sleep through the night. And French parents are more distressed when a baby fails to meet this expectation. Expectations inform choices. I highly suspect that French parents are more likely to put the baby to sleep in another room and more likely to ignore the little groans and whimpers that, if not reinforced, will often go away. The little noises and even short spells of crying are necessarily part of the process by which a baby learns to self-soothe (Ferber 2006). Empirical research clearly shows that *how* parents put babies to sleep (awake, on their back, not with a bottle, and not breastfeeding) does make a difference in the child's development and particularly in their risk for developing depression later in life (Paulson, Dauber, and Leiferman 2006). This is probably because sleep plays such a huge part in the development of depression and good sleep habits can begin in infancy.

The American Academy of Pediatrics offers some very useful guidelines developed in our culture, for our culture. Although we do live in a heterogeneous society with many different philosophies and folkways concerning infant care and child rearing, we are also in a unique position in history to have a well researched scientific basis for many of our practices—the practices that matter the most to long-term psychological adjustment and physical health. While much ambiguity still exists and will continue to exist, neither are we cast adrift on an ocean of uncertainty. In past times and in primitive societies the illusion of certainty was maintained through custom, ritual, and the prescribed roles of shaman, witch doctor, wise woman, and prophetess. In today's world we have less certainty in one sense but more certainty in another. What information we do have is based on science, and although science does change over time, it offers a much more solid footing than superstition. In our world the shaman, witch doctor, wise woman, and prophetess have been replaced by medical professionals—pediatricians, psychologists, educators, and social workers.

A great benefit of our science-based culture is that, when you feel overwhelmed by parenting, you can consult someone who has studied and specialized in the issues that concern you. You are not alone. Nor are the anxieties of our modern times altogether different from those of "modern times" almost a century ago. Consider this passage, penned in 1922 and published in the popular magazine *Good Housekeeping*: "Under the best of condition, it is a solemn and hazardous business, bringing up our precious children; but it is no longer a black forest without a compass or a path. We have only made a beginning; we all know in our hearts how we fail; how over and over, we fail. We probably are doing things to our children as wrong and foolish as our grandmothers did. But at least we know a little more than they which is the path for us to follow; and to find in the black forest we have a compass if we will only learn how to use it" (Fisher 1922, 172). The "compass" that Dorothy Fisher refers to in this passage is science. And science suggests that when it comes to sleeping, it is best for baby to learn early how to settle herself to sleep.

What About Feeding?

Different choices often have differing emotional costs, and this is very true when it comes to parenting. There are financial costs associated with going back to work and putting the child in day care, and there are financial costs involved in quitting work and staying home to raise a baby. But there are emotional costs to each of these choices as well. While the financial costs might be the same for two different people with similar incomes and similar child-care costs and needs, the emotional costs and rewards of various choices vary tremendously across individuals.

Consider breastfeeding. For some women, nursing is easy and natural. Science has shown over and again that the breast is "better" than the bottle in many ways—imparting benefits to the infant's developing immune system and providing deep psychological comforts of skin-to-skin contact and proximity to the mother's familiar heartbeat. But for a woman who must return to work soon after giving birth, for a woman whose identity is defined by her commitment to professional pursuits, for a woman who can't nurse, or for a woman who doesn't like nursing, the choice of breastfeeding may exact too high a toll. Artful living means living within one's means—both emotionally and financially. A Lexus may be better than a Kia, but if you can't afford a Lexus, a Kia will get you around town quite readily.

Blair made an appointment with me after her second child was born because she had gotten terribly depressed after the first baby. For her first child, she had prepared for a natural childbirth but ended up with an emergency C-section. As a result, she came home from the hospital feeling like a failure. She had nursed for eight months but found it exhausting. She resented the baby and wondered if she was a bad mother. She had been on meds until she got pregnant and went off them against medical advice.

For her second baby, Blair has decided to bottlefeed, and she's trying a quasi schedule—not too rigid but not on demand either. This time she's trying to use more helpful thinking patterns than she did with her first baby. She's learning to identify and change her global thinking and to distinguish between what she does and does not have control over. She's also learning that it's more than okay to let her children tolerate a little distress. In psychology, the standard we're aiming for is "good enough" parenting. Being the best is a myth, and the sooner you let go of it the sooner you'll be tolerating ambiguity gracefully and doing the best you can. Like Blair, you might even begin to enjoy parenting.

Reasonable vs. Unreasonable Guilt

Diane Ehrensaft, child psychologist and author of *Spoiling Childhood: How Well-Meaning Parents Are Giving Children Too Much—But Not What They Need*, observes that guilt is the overriding theme of modern American parenthood: "We parent like Tarzan on a rope, wildly swinging from never being there enough to being there far too much. It is time to find the key to the following riddle: How does this generation of parents simultaneously get construed as putting their own needs first and accused of being overly focused on their children? The answer to the riddle is one word—guilt" (Ehrensaft

1997, 74). The helicopter parent gives way to the two-martini parent and the result is dizzying (Belkin 2009).

Developing the ability to distinguish between what one can and cannot control is the very essence of learning to tolerate ambiguity gracefully; it is also the key to distinguishing between reasonable and unreasonable guilt. Guilt is a very useful emotion that can alert you to personal and social transgressions. Guilt lets you know when you've hurt someone so that you can make amends and repair relationships. Guilt lets you know when you've broken trust with yourself or violated your own integrity. The feeling of guilt lets you know you can get back on track and become the person you want to be. But guilt can also be a tyrant. You *may* have control over whether you breastfeed or bottle-feed or use some combination of both. You do *not* have control over whether your baby prefers one or the other or whether your baby "spits you out" at six months, the way Margaret's son Will did.

Margaret was terribly hurt and felt like a failure. But her second child, daughter Cameron, more than made up for Will's "rejection." She nursed Cameron for two years and felt very successful. But eventually she had to admit that she probably had little to do with Will's preference for the bottle. Will continued to be active and stridently independent all the way into manhood, and Cameron is still much different from her brother. You may have control over whether you feed on demand or you use a schedule of some sort (and there are many variations to choose from). But you don't necessarily have control over what works. You don't have control over whether or when your baby sleeps through the night, but you do have control over whether you put him to sleep in his own bed, on his back, awake, and without a bottle. You don't have control over how intelligent your child is or how successful she becomes, but you do have control over whether you read to her, sing to her, tickle her, and play with her. These distinctions are important and helpful in learning to navigate the minefield of uncertainties and enjoy parenting. Otherwise, guilt can very easily rob you of joy.

If you feel guilty, it might mean that you have good reason to be. But that depends. When guilt is merited, it is simply a *signal to change something*. When guilt is warranted, the solution is simple, even if it is not always pleasant. Pay attention to the guilt. By tuning in to these feelings instead of stuffing them or wallowing in them, you can be honest with yourself and change what needs to be changed. I know that's easier said than done, but it is nonetheless true. If you can't change whatever it is on your own, then get help. And if you can't change it because it's in the past, then the only reasonable thing to do is forgive yourself and let it go. The litmus test, once again, involves being able to distinguish clearly between what you do have control over and what you do not. Two things you do *not* need to feel guilty about are teaching your child to tolerate a little distress and sending your child to day care.

Filling in the Blanks

Ambiguity, not knowing, is very anxiety provoking (Gilbert 2009). No one likes to feel anxious, so we usually have some coping strategies to help us either avoid or deal with anxiety. A common coping strategy to help us manage the anxiety of not knowing is to try to eliminate it. When we're faced with ambiguity, when we don't know the reasons or the outcome, we often fill in the blanks with conjecture. Much of the time, speculation is projection, meaning that we project what we *fear* into the future or onto others.

Speculating about "why" is usually futile. Filling in the blanks with blanket statements about what kind of person a particular incident means you "really are" is worse than useless. It is the global thinking, the permanent, pervasive, personal attributions for negative events that characterizes all depressions (Seligman 1990). Global thinking, negative thinking, generates neurotransmitters that suck up serotonin while increasing cortisol and other stress hormones. It is this sort of erroneous, global conclusion that often drives a mom or dad to withdraw from the parenting role, and it is the *recoil* from involvement with the infant that is most damaging to the baby.

The Importance of Involved Dads

A national study of children and their parents is underway, called the Early Childhood Longitudinal Study. Longitudinal studies are rare because they are expensive and they collect data over a very long period of time. This study has enrolled 5,089 two-parent families, and the first "waves" of data have begun to come in.

James F. Paulson, Ph.D., from the Center for Pediatric Research heads up one group that is looking at the data. Data collected at nine months and at twenty-four months into the study confirm the incidence rate of postpartum depression is 14 percent for mothers and 10 percent for fathers (Paulson, Dauber, and Leiferman 2006). One of the most interesting findings of this study centers around parental depression. According to the data, a depressed parent is much more likely to withdraw from interacting with the baby. When either the mother or the father or both are depressed, the depressed parent is less likely to read, sing, or tell stories to the baby. Traditionally, some may have thought that a father's withdrawal from the baby would be less damaging than if a child's mother withdrew. But the data from the Early Childhood Longitudinal Study shows how important a father's involvement can be. In fact, the data shows that fathers play an important role in the baby's language development (Paulson, Keefe, and Leiferman 2009). So, if you're a dad who is struggling, perhaps feeling displaced or resentful, and these painful feelings prompt you to withdraw from your newborn, please think again. And if you just can't pull yourself out of your funk by your bootstraps, by all means, get some help. That baby needs you even now, whether it feels that way to you or not.

Managing Expectations

Americans are often accused by people from other cultures of having difficulty distinguishing between wants and needs—our own as well as our children's. And they may sometimes be right. Feeling guilty will inevitably lead to overcompensating, and overcompensating will eventually lead to resentment—and there you have the oscillations. Guilt can impel parents to confuse the best interests of the child with getting the best there is, choosing the most expensive, the most comfortable, or "anything the she wants." If you feel guilty or if you find yourself swinging between being too involved and not being involved enough, please get professional help. If you can't tell the difference between overinvolvement and underinvolvement, a therapist will also do you good. Maybe you need to make radical changes in your life and your work, but maybe you need to change your expectations. A professional who is well versed in these issues and who can offer an objective view can provide you with the perspective you may be missing.

Brady planned her pregnancy and the birth of her child very thoroughly, including drawing up a birth plan and hiring a doula to help. With all of her careful planning, she was also one of the women for whom everything seemed to go wrong. It all started when her water broke but labor did not follow. She was admitted to the hospital and given pitosin to induce labor. Then her contractions still didn't come and the pitosin was increased. When she finally did start to contract, she was already tired and the contractions were hard but not very productive. She begged for an epidural, something she never thought she'd want. After making this concession to her own comfort, it seemed almost insulting that the epidural had no noticeable effect. Finally Brady was given stadol, which made her "not care" that the contractions were painful, even though she still felt them and still experienced them as painful.

When it was finally time to push, Brady worked mightily for three hours despite already being exhausted. But Nikki, a big baby girl, got stuck in the birth canal. Brady knew she was in trouble when the nurse-midwife paged the on-call doctor. They did eventually extricate the baby without need of a C-section, but a nerve to her right hand and shoulder was damaged in the struggle. Not having the birth she had envisioned, Brady felt like a bad mother and a failure.

During our first session I had identified her overly global, black-and-white thinking and helped her see her experience with more nuance. She left this session feeling optimistic and empowered. With this newfound perspective and optimism, she decided to stop allowing her baby girl to chew on her sore nipples (she had been indulging the baby as a way of compensating for what she thought of as her previous failure). Brady decided to train Nikki to work her chewing impulse out on a pacifier instead.

In the next session she related the story: Since she had heard that babies will sometimes take the pacifier if it has something sweet on it, she looked for some sugar in her pantry. Out of sugar, she used honey instead. And as she told the story, her tears started to flow. She had given her tiny baby daughter honey without knowing that honey can cause infant botulism poisoning. Her interpretation: "I almost killed my baby."

I pointed out that she made a judgment call that she later found out was less than optimal, and when she found out she changed her strategy. That is a learning curve. You start with a guess, do the best you can, and observe the results or get new information. Then you can change your approach, try again, again observe the results, take in the information, adjust what you do, and keep trying until you hit upon something that works. Learning curves are graphed as a function of success over time. And it can take a thousand repetitions to become proficient at just about anything—including parenting (Gladwell 2008).

I asked Brady if the baby had been in the ICU. She hadn't. I asked how many times she had coded and needed to be resuscitated. None. Global thinking leads to assuming that the worst will happen, and this tendency interferes with learning. I went on to work with Brady on the cognitive distortions that characterized her depression, pointing out how quickly her mind went from putting the tiniest bit of honey on her daughter's pacifier to the fantasy of being dragged away from her child's gravesite for eternal lockup as a bad mom. The more I exaggerated, the calmer Brady became. She breathed a deep sigh of relief, threw her head back, and asked how she could *ever* change her thinking. "Well," I replied, "to change your thinking you'll need to really *embrace the learning curve*. By the time you have ten thousand repetitions, you'll be an expert." She laughed.

Brady continued to struggle with her global thinking for several more sessions, and I continued to educate her about how to experience her emotions, detach from them, validate them, and put them into perspective. Eventually she got used to the process of catching herself "going global" and calming herself by challenging her thinking to be more specific, more nuanced, and more self-accepting. Eventually she grew confident that her love for Nikki would guide her observations and *inform* her learning curve. Brady began to feel that the rest of her life with Nikki will be a long, wonderful journey of learning, doing the best she can, and letting go of the things she can't control. Embracing the journey of discovery makes it more pleasurable.

Adoption, Parenting Issues, and Depression

Brady is a typical postpartum depression patient. Her depression has all the same cognitive distortions that every other garden-variety depression has, but it's framed as a pathological response to the hormones of pregnancy and the drop in those hormones that occur after delivery (Bloch et al. 2000). The hormonal frame joins with the mother's global thinking to create an overall sense of failure as a mother, snowballing to prompt a desire to recoil from the parenting role.

But, as we've seen, fathers also experience depression and may also tend to conclude erroneously that they just aren't good at being a dad. And the same thing can happen to adoptive parents, who can also experience depression. Parenting choices for the adoptive parent can be especially fraught, particularly if they constantly contrast their experience with what they consider a "normal" route to parenting. Thus, just as biological parents can experience guilt and depression because of difficult parenting issues, so too can those who adopt. And adoptive parents have the challenge of wondering if delayed or effortful attachment to their new baby means that they weren't "meant" to be parents, that the adoption was a mistake.

Myers and Whitney had their first child the usual way—from conception to unmedicated delivery, their son's arrival conformed to cultural expectations of what is "normal," and it was relatively easy. Whitney breastfed and enjoyed motherhood, so she logically expected the second time around to be pretty much the same. It wasn't. She had a very difficult second labor and ended up with an emergency C-section. The baby was in the N-ICU for several weeks. Whitney felt like a failure and had a bad case of postpartum depression. That depression was so horrible that she never wanted to go through anything like it again. But Myers and Whitney wanted a third child.

Believing that the postpartum depression Whitney had experienced was hormonal, they adopted. Myers and Whitney had both loved their Peace Corps experiences in Peru, so it seemed fitting to adopt a Peruvian child, native of a land they felt so warmly toward. Unlike many international adoptions, their adoption process went smoothly and relatively quickly. But about 15 percent of adoptive parents go through clinical depression after the baby arrives (Senecky et al. 2009). However, adoptive parents don't have the hormones to explain away their feelings, and fewer adoptive parents are depressed after baby than before, when they were going through all the infertility and all the uncertainty (Senecky et al. 2009).

Myers and Whitney didn't need to grieve infertility because they had chosen to adopt despite being able to get pregnant. But couples who have gone through infertility, who have experienced the medicalization of conception or the multiple, repeated, devastating losses that eventuate in adoption, these parents often find themselves grieving just when they expect to be welcoming. Even though their situation was different from that of the "typical" adoptive couple, they still were vulnerable to the pitfall of unevaluated expectations, which can affect all parents, adoptive or not.

Myers and Whitney didn't expect that the attachment process would be different or more difficult. They didn't expect that getting up in the middle of the night would be more annoying. They didn't expect their other children to protest, act out, and become difficult. They didn't expect a lot of things. When the unexpected challenges and unforeseen emotions hit Myers and Whitney, they wondered what these surprise emotions might mean. Were they bad parents? Had they gotten a bad kid? Were they too old to be parenting a baby? Not knowing, they began to fill in the blanks with speculation. Myers and Whitney *both* tanked into clinical depression.

Coping Strategies

There are some specific coping strategies that work well when you're doing the work of parenting. As you face your day, babe in arms, try to begin practicing some of these effective strategies to help you meet challenges with more equilibrium.

Unhooking Mood from Behavior

Compartmentalizing your emotions means that you put your emotions aside and do what you need to do—just because. Just because you want to be the best parent that you can be at this moment, you hit the pause button on your exhaustion and tears and chatter to a baby who cannot understand your words. Just because you know it's better for the baby, you do the hard thing and put her down on her back in her own bed and leave the room.

The first rule of life is this: if you can't make it better, at least don't make it worse. Because you want things to be better, you don't make them worse. Because you want to love your baby son, you read to him. You may be sick to death of his board books, but you want to help his eventual language development, so you read the book anyway. Because you want to like being a mommy (or daddy) you smile—even if it's an insincere, plastic, half smile. Research shows that using the facial muscles involved in smiling to smile when you don't feel like it can actually help you shift your emotions (Papa and Bonanno 2008). You wish you felt better, so you sing. You sing, and you sing, and you sing. You sing to your baby and don't worry about whether the neighbors would vote you off the island. Because when you can't make it better, you do things that at least don't make it worse—and singing sometimes actually surprises you by making you feel better (Blood and Zatorre 2001).

There is a place for the old adage "fake it 'til you make it." Sometimes when you love, when you parent, you have to fake it. And you fake it until you don't have to fake anymore. Will it be hard? Yes. It will feel hard, super hard, for a little while—while you're depressed. But no emotion lasts forever (Gross 1998). And every time you separate your behavior from your feelings, every time you do the hard thing, you are gaining a little bit of control over your emotions and getting a little bit stronger. Every time you catch yourself "going global" and pull your mind back to the present, every time you exercise your choice to just deal with what is as it is at *this* moment in time, you gain a little more control. Little by little, step by step, one day, one moment at a time, you gain control over this mood state that feels so overwhelming and so dark. Just because you want to find some little thing you can have control over, you make yourself think about what life will be like when it's better. And soon you discover that your attention is like a muscle—little by little, one thought at a time, you develop the capacity to control where your attention goes. The past is unchangeable and the future is unknowable. Keep your mind away from what is unchangeable; do not allow yourself to speculate about what is unknowable. Just for now—just because—stay in the present moment and deal as best you can.

A Word About Colic

Colic is a tough row to hoe, so I want to give it a special mention in this coping-skills section. You may do a lot of coping (rather than feeling joyful) in the first weeks if you happen to get a colicky baby. That's okay. It will be hard, but you can do it. As with most things, it's good to have accurate information at hand and patience with yourself in your heart.

The old nature-versus-nurture debate has been resolved—both are important; neither stands alone. But most surprisingly, and perhaps hardest to grasp, is that influence is *reciprocal*. The baby is not a *tabula rasa*, an unformatted disk. The baby comes preprogrammed in ways that you will react to as well as influence (Bell and Belsky 2008; Dix 1991). This may be especially important when it comes to colic.

You are likely to respond differently to a high-reactive baby than you would if your baby were low reactive. Babies who are difficult to soothe are frustrating. One study showed that more than 91 percent of mothers with a colicky infant experienced tension in the marriage and disruption in their social relationships as a result of the baby's colic (Levitski and Cooper 2000). Wow! That's a lot of power for a little person to wield. It's hard for others to be around a crying, screaming infant, and they tend to look to the mother to be able to soothe her baby. No wonder mothers feel blamed and pressured to attain an unattainable perfection.

You get to have your feelings. You get to experience them—like waves of the ocean crashing on the shore. Later, they will recede again. You get to look at them—an attitude of curiosity always helps. You get to name them out loud. In some cultures, emotions are considered to be demons that can have control only when they are unnamed. But I've found that as soon as emotions are known and named—poof! They lose some of their power and intensity. You just don't get to act on them. Emotions are not "Truth" with a capital T. Emotions are true of your experience in *this* moment, and that is all. At this moment, all the energy is going out and there isn't much coming back to you in the way of positive reinforcement. But it won't always be this way.

Babies change daily, weekly, monthly. Go ahead and take a moment to fantasize. Fantasize about taking a one-way cruise to the Caribbean, running away to join a hippie commune in Hawaii, or going to work in a diner in Wisconsin while training to be a professional ice skater. But remember, this is your imagination, so while you're at it, allow yourself to also fantasize about a time when things will be better—perhaps about holding your two-year-old by the hand while she walks proudly up to her day-care center. Once inside, she eagerly hugs her new best friend, dismissing you with "It's okay, Mommy. You can go now." And when you've had your moment of reverie, return to the present, focus on where you are and what you're doing now, breathe slowly and deeply, and stay emotionally connected. You did not cause the crying, but you do respond to it. Respond; don't react. Sometimes you can find something to do that helps; sometimes not. Either way, you soon learn that parenting is a two-way street, and managing your own anxieties, getting comfortable being uncomfortable, is one of the best things you can do for yourself and, ultimately, for the baby.

Mindfulness: Living in the Present Moment

The baby changes every day. The baby learns to focus. The baby learns to control his muscles—he reaches out to grab the toy dangling over his carrier. Yesterday she was frustrated because she tried and couldn't get her mind and her body to do what she was concentrating so hard on. It's fascinating to watch a baby learn. You can almost see the little wheels turning. You can see the effort, the strain. Today he got it. You can see how much delight there is for him in trying so hard and finally getting it.

You change every day. You learn to focus. You learn to control your attention and redirect your thoughts. Yesterday you were frustrated because you tried and couldn't, but today you might get it. If not today, perhaps tomorrow. Have you forgotten how good it feels to try hard to do something and finally get it? Tomorrow is a different day. Wonder what the baby will learn today. Wonder what you will learn today. Journal each day's triumphs—but only the triumphs.

Learning to stay in the present moment, to do one thing at a time and to be emotionally present to each and every thing you do, is a wonderful antidote to depression and an essential and often overlooked key to happiness (Brown and Ryan 2003). Our culture seems to insist that multitasking is a skill and is necessary for success in meeting the many demands of our modern lives. But multitasking is a myth—and a really dangerous one. Recent research shows that, while multitaskers might *feel* efficient in the short run, they actually are worse at just about everything. Multitaskers don't focus as well as non-multitaskers; they're more distractible and weaker at shifting from one task to another and at organizing information (Ophir, Nass, and Wagner 2009; Crenshaw 2008).

The opposite of multitasking is mindfulness. *Mindfulness* is the capacity to be entirely present—mind, body, and emotions—in the present moment, to give one's full and undivided attention to one thing at a time. The term "mindfulness" is borrowed from Buddhism, but it has a counterpart in Christianity. The Christian tradition knows mindfulness variously as contemplative prayer or "the practice of the presence of God" (Lawrence and Smith 1897). Protestant Christians know it as "abiding in Christ" (Murray 2003). The idea behind these terms is precisely that everything a person does is of equal value and ought to be done when mentally, emotionally, and spiritually present. Another way to phrase it is to say that being fully present in the moment allows one to be "recollected," or aware that everything one does, one does in the presence of God. Thus, to live a life recollected to the presence of God is to live in sacred time. Babies live in the moment and need the full and undivided attention of their caretakers. Babies experience this full and undivided attention as love.

Mindfulness has very tangible benefits to health and well-being. Several studies show that the benefits of mindfulness, meditation, or self-hypnosis include real changes to the brain—positive changes to the same areas of the brain that show damage in people who have experienced prolonged stress, anxiety, or depression (Lutz et al. 2004; Lazar et al. 2005). Mindfulness-based cognitive behavioral therapy for depression has also been shown repeatedly to be highly effective in preventing relapse (Teasdale et al. 2000; Williams et al. 2000), as has hypnosis (Yapko 2001b). One major weakness of medications in the treatment of depression is that they have a high relapse rate (Evans et al. 1992).

Parenthood, the Passionate Dance

"Passion" comes from the Greek root word *pathos*, which means "to suffer." The words "patient" and "patience" also both come from this root word. Thus, to be patient means to suffer delays. To exercise patience means to suffer the frustration of failures.

To be passionate about life, we must be willing to suffer delays of gratification and the many frustrations involved in learning. We must be willing to suffer the disappointment of finding that life does not meet our expectations, the discomfort of adjusting our expectations to conform to reality rather than insisting that reality conform to our expectations. To be passionate about life, we must be willing to suffer the discomfort of uncertainty—to get comfortable being uncomfortable. And parenthood, like the passionate Argentine tango, is an improvisational dance. You can go to a franchise dance studio and learn some dance steps, but it won't be the Argentine tango. The steps are as basic as walking, but the complexity comes in the connection and the need for each partner to hold their own balance. Likewise, you can read some parenting books and follow the latest parenting trends; but unless you've got the connection, you're not dancing—you're doing steps. Parenthood, like the tango, is a passionate dance.

Exercises for Chapter 6

Exercise 1: Noticing

Training yourself to notice things in a new way is a matter of paying attention. Most of us favor one sensory modality over the others, and until we try to pay attention to another modality we don't know what we've been missing. So I'm going to give you a couple of ideas for each sense; but in order to really challenge yourself to grow in a whole new way, you'll have to think of a few more that are particular to you.

Sight

* Sit in a park or some other nature spot with your notebook and note twenty-five different living things (animal or insect).

* Go to a public place you've never been before and stand in the entrance. Stay a little out of the way of people coming and going. Pause and look around, taking in all the sights. Divide your notebook page into two columns. Jot down everything you see, one item per line. Then in the other column, jot down how each thing makes you feel. Be specific.

Sound

- Go to a park or some other nature spot with your notebook and find a comfortable place to sit. Close your eyes and challenge yourself to identify twenty-five different sounds.

- Go to a public place with lots of people, somewhere you can sit comfortably with your notebook (train stations are good for this exercise). Close your eyes and try to identify twenty-five different sounds. Jot them down in your notebook.

Touch

- Gather twenty-five different objects with different textures (for example, a chamois, a silk scarf, a loofah, some suede, cotton, linen, or terrycloth, a piece of rubber, a feather, microfiber, nylon, wool, and so on). Place them in a box, and with your eyes closed, identify each one. A variation of this exercise is to have your partner or a friend touch you with each object randomly and as you guess. It could even be more interesting if someone else picked the objects and you had to identify them by touch alone.

- Get a bag of mixed beans (they sell these for soups). Open the bag and empty all the beans into a large box or bowl. Blindfold yourself and sort the beans into piles according to size and shape—the navy beans in one pile, lentils in another, the fava beans another, and the butter beans another. Challenge yourself to sort through all the beans before taking the blindfold off.

Taste

- Take a wine- or coffee-tasting class. Take notes on each taste discrimination you learn. Notice that in these classes you don't necessarily swallow; rather, you swill, smell, swish, and spit.

- Make up your own tasting task: get about seven of whatever it is you want to learn to develop fine discriminations for—chocolate, herb teas, whatever. Line them up in front of you. Taste one slowly and carefully, writing down your impressions and your emotions in your notebook. Cleanse your palate before moving on to the next item.

Smell

- Visit a perfume factory or cigar shop. Try to identify the different elements of each fragrance.

- Pick a few leaves or blades of grass. Crush them and inhale the green aroma notes.

- Line up about five different jars of spices in front of you, keeping the lids on until you're ready to smell. Open one bottle and inhale gently. Close it again. Cleanse your nose by blowing a little air through it quickly, like panting with your mouth closed. Repeat with the next spice. Go back and forth between two until you can distinguish them clearly before moving on to the next.

Kinesthetic

The kinesthetic "sense" is really not a sense at all but the coordination of several senses for determining your position in space. Ordinarily your brain takes in auditory and visual information (and sometimes touch) to calibrate your movements and orient the position of your body. But if you close your eyes, you withdraw one source of external information and have to focus on your own body's internal cues. (This is called *proprioception,* meaning "one's own" perception.)

- Stand on one foot until you are well balanced. Now close your eyes. Write down what you noticed about this exercise.

- At your local health club locate a bosu—a rubber half ball or dome on a firm platform. Flip the bosu over so that platform faces up, and sit on it, balancing yourself on the domed portion. Once you've situated yourself, move your torso gently in a circle and feel the balance point in your body. Now close your eyes, focus internally, and again move your torso gently in a circle while trying to maintain balance.

Exercise 2: Setting Standards

We all have the same amount of time—twenty-four hours in a day—of which we need about eight to sleep. We have differing amounts of emotional and financial resources to allocate to those remaining sixteen hours. That means that we cannot possibly do all things equally well or aspire to a standard of excellence in everything unless we limit our commitments. This necessitates making some clear-eyed decisions about which activities we will pitch to a standard of excellence, which we will pitch to a "make do" standard, and which we will pitch to a "get by" standard.

What I'd like you to do is to sit down with your notebook and write down all the major roles you occupy in life: mother/father, spouse, child, employee, supervisor, and so on. Next, list several tasks that you have to perform in each role, and assign each task a priority rating. This rating needs to be an honest estimate of what standard you will aspire to for that task—excellence, middling, or getting by. Challenge yourself to really be honest.

Exercise 3: Determining Degrees of Influence

This exercise involves estimating the degree of influence you have over various outcomes. With your notebook in hand, I'd like for you to list several outcomes that are really important to you. These might include things like paying off a credit card, getting out of debt, finishing a degree, putting the final touches on a pet project, painting a room, folding three loads of laundry, getting someone you love to stop drinking, getting someone to bring a salad to your potluck, changing the oil in your car, or any number of other things. Be sure to include some things that involve your own behavior (like painting, folding, and so on) and some things that involve someone else complying with a request you make (agreeing, following through).

It will help if you construct the list in two columns—one for the outcome you desire and the other for your estimate of how much influence you have over that outcome. When you have your list, go through and assign a numeric value to your estimate of your influence. You might want to compare your list and your ratings with the list that your partner or friend generated. Now ask yourself whether there might be objective ways to verify some of your estimates. For example, winning the lottery will carry with it a low probability if you buy a ticket and a zero probability if you don't buy a ticket.

If any of your behaviors are rated 100 percent, think again. How many unforeseen circumstances beyond your influence could derail you? Even picking up the phone and dialing depends on the weather in some places.

If any behaviors involving another person are rated more than 50 percent, think again. You are only 50 percent of any interaction, so the very most you can possibly contribute is half, even if you are an excellent communicator and fabulously persuasive.

CHAPTER 7

Money: Beyond Smoke and Mirrors

Choose the life that is most useful, and habit will make it the most agreeable.

Sir Francis Bacon

My mother grew up in Eastern Kentucky during the Great Depression. Back in the hollers of Eastern Kentucky folks had a saying: "Love flies out the window when poverty walks through the door." Of course, from everything I can tell, just about everyone was poor by our standards in that place at that time, but not everyone knew it. Not everyone felt poor. And the ones who didn't feel poor were the ones who managed what few resources they had well. Mother only got one pair of shoes a year—in the fall when school started up. And that meant that by summer she, and most of the kids she knew, went barefoot, just like in all those Norman Rockwell paintings. Whatever your economic circumstances, you can feel rich or poor depending on how you manage your expectations and your resources, and managing your finances well is one of the best things you can do to protect your relationship.

Money Illusions

Economists have long known that people are not logical or rational when it comes to money. The concept of "money illusion" is attributed to Miles Maynard Keynes and made famous (at least among economists) by Irvin Fisher's book of the same name (Fisher 1928). The phrase refers to people's tendency to think about money in terms of its face value instead of purchasing power (Shafir, Diamond, and Tversky 1997). This illusion leads people to spend more when they are using credit cards than when they're using cash (Feinberg 1986; Hirschman 1979; Prelec and Simester 2001) and to have inaccurate mental categories about how much money they have or owe (Prelec and Loewenstein 1998). Neuroscientists have even identified the area of the brain (the medial prefrontal cortex) that is involved in money illusion (Weber et al. 2009). Marketing tactics exploit money illusion when they charge the same for something but make the item smaller, when they devise "pennies-a-day" schemes, or by urging you to think about purchases as investments (Gourville 1998).

The money illusion is directly related to depression because it fosters poor choices, and those choices have repercussions. Stuck in a financial rut, people subject to the money illusion are susceptible to low self-confidence, an external locus of control, and pessimistic expectations about life. A study aimed at profiling people who got into difficulty with credit found that "unsuccessful credit users displayed greater external locus of control, lower self-efficacy, viewed money as a source of power and prestige, took fewer steps to retain their money, displayed lower risk-taking and sensation-seeking tendencies, and expressed greater anxiety about financial matters than successful users" (Tokunaga 1993, 285). So, this group demonstrated behaviors and attitudes that fit right into the cognitive styles we know make one vulnerable to depression—an external locus of control, low feelings of self-efficacy coupled with carelessness with money on one hand and fearfulness on the other. And these cognitive risk factors contributed to creating tricky financial problems that they were ill-equipped to solve (another risk factor for depression).

Financial Trouble and Your Health

Financial distress and low socioeconomic status are stressors, and they have long been known to be important factors for all kinds of medical problems including depression and suicide (Collier 2009; Noh 2009; Kumar et al. 1996). Intuitively, we all know that financial difficulties can strain a marriage, and even before the economic downturn of recent years, research had shown that money problems can be a risk factor for postpartum depression (Beck 2001; Escriba et al. 1999; Segre et al. 2007). Having children changes everything in a couple's life, including finances. That's why I'm wrapping up this book with a chapter dedicated to negotiating your new financial terrain. Remaining open to this information may seem scary at first, but I encourage you to do so. The information you find here will help reduce the amount of ambiguity you have to deal with, allowing you to get a handle on your illusions and develop structures to avoid the common pitfalls that can cause money-induced stress, relationship conflict, and depression.

One Couple's Financial Journey

You may be well aware of the financial impact of parenthood, or you may be just beginning to think about it. Because the subject is pretty complex, it's helpful to see how another couple experiences these changes. Let's take a close look at Taylor and Jody to see how their new financial situation surprised them. We'll be following them throughout the chapter.

Taylor and Jody had opted to defer childbearing until they had set a firm financial base and were established in their careers. But seven years of infertility treatments, including several rounds of in-vitro fertilization, drained their savings. They were ecstatic that the treatments ultimately met with success, but they faced parenthood without the nest egg they had hoped to have.

After Miles was born, Jody opted to stay home to take care of him while Taylor continued to climb the corporate ladder. Jody envisioned herself working at home on various projects, some that would generate income and others that were just necessary to keep life running smoothly. She could see it vividly: her perfectly compliant infant would nurse contentedly, bundle easily, and carry effortlessly, cooing comfortably in his carrier. Women in other cultures returned to the fields with their babies in slings, so why shouldn't Jody?

But life at home with the new baby was not the picture of maternal bliss that Jody had imagined. It started to seem inevitable that Miles would have a messy poop (requiring Jody to change Miles and herself) just as Jody was stepping out the door. This was especially frustrating when Jody was dressed up for a business appointment, as was often the case. Or Miles would spit up. Or he would wail inconsolably. The sources of the delays were as unpredictable as they were frustrating.

Meanwhile, Taylor missed being with the baby and sometimes resented that Jody "got" to stay home full-time; work did not feel like a privilege to him. With their new lack of liquidity, Taylor felt even more pressure to work hard to produce. He and Jody hadn't foreseen just how much a new baby could challenge their finances, and the stress began to wear on them. Whatever illusory budget they had was based on Taylor's salary alone, and Taylor held a tight rein, his grip a mixture of anxiety and entitlement. Taylor complained about Jody's spending, since, as he saw it, she was the one at home making most of the purchases. Jody felt unjustly criticized and wondered what impostor had replaced her fun-loving, risk-taking partner. She didn't like feeling defensive or having to justify what she spent on diapers—a necessity—not to mention that sometimes she resorted to a babysitter just so she could do the work that would benefit both of them. She felt as though her indulgences were few—certainly fewer than Taylor's! Only rarely did she get a babysitter so she could go out with the girls, and she considered these reasonable breaks that helped her maintain her adult identity and some semblance of sanity. But the disharmony ate away at their formerly affectionate and collaborative partnership.

By the time they came to me, I could see that both Taylor and Jody lived with some level of depression. Although Jody freely made the choice to stay home with the baby, putting her career on hold for a while, both she and Taylor had trouble valuing her contribution to the family when it didn't have a dollar amount attached. And without Jody's income, their finances were more fuzzy and less predictable than they had once been. This set up an unpleasant cycle involving arguments about money (surprises and disappointments abound when uncertainty rules the day), defensiveness on Jody's part, and bouts of trading blame between the two of them.

Strategies and Tactics

Although the particulars of Jody and Taylor's finances might be different from other couples, the pattern of their arguments was as common as lint. The path out of the maze was also fairly common: find ways to value intangible contributions (making the intangible tangible, using money if necessary), and contain unpredictability as much as possible in order to stop the blame game. Once these criteria are met, it's possible to talk openly and honestly about feelings—hopes and dreams and how each person misses the other, even though they love their new life.

When facing problems, it's often helpful to first define a goal and then choose the strategies and tactics that will be most helpful in achieving the goal. Basic financial goals start with survival and gradually increase to include savings and planning for the future. Given that financial strains often make the difference between a harmonious relationship and a union torn asunder by strife, it makes sense to work toward a well-thought-out, mutually agreed-upon approach with your partner, a plan that includes methods for achieving clearly defined financial goals and staying out of marital therapy. Let's explore the elements of this approach.

Separate Mood from Behavior

We've looked at this tactic before, and it applies just as much when you're working with finances. After all, moods that you act on can have a significant impact on your financial situation. Complicating matters further is the fact that people who are depressed often allow their moods to enslave their behavior. For example, Jody no longer followed a routine or planned her day in advance. Instead she hoped she would feel up to making calls, running errands, balancing the checkbook, or doing housework and laundry. She often didn't feel like cooking, so she reached for the phone, ordering carryout for Taylor to pick up on his way home from work—a real source of friction and resentment when he paid the tab.

For his part, Taylor would justify getting in the car at lunchtime to visit his local fast-food joint or greasy spoon, simply because he hadn't felt like fixing a sandwich or grabbing an apple and granola bar on the way out the door in the morning. Of course, Taylor's budgetary transgressions didn't surface until he and Jody started implementing their family meetings—but I get ahead of myself. It's not that ordering carryout is a terrible thing. But ordering carryout because the *mood* wasn't there to cook is counterproductive on many levels. So, learning to decouple mood from behavior is often a top priority in treating depression. There is a time and place for everything—a time to be internally oriented to your own thoughts and feelings and a time to be externally oriented to the goals and objectives you have.

This is a very important principle. Think about other successes you've had in life. You didn't get a high-school diploma or a college degree by going to class only when you felt like it; you accomplished those milestones in life by doing what the situation demanded despite whatever you might have been feeling. And some days were easier than others—that's life.

When you're struggling with strong emotions or demands that exceed your emotional resources, you can most easily unplug your behavior from your mood by first putting as many behaviors as possible on autopilot, subjecting as many acts as possible to ritual, routine, or rhythm. Even as I recommend ritual, routine, and rhythm, I want to caution against interpreting this too rigidly. My rule of thumb is to increase structure when chaos increases and to lighten up when there is more order. In other words, we're aiming for a balance of structure and flexibility. When structure is too rigid and budgets are too tight, the buildup of tension inevitably leads to a fall. There has to be some room for the small splurge and the enjoyment of spontaneity, because a completely automatic life is dull and lacking in vibrancy. Again, it's not that the occasional visit to Starbucks or Mickey D's is a terrible thing, but we must corral such romps so that they don't overrun a carefully crafted spending plan. Room must also be left for measured spontaneity—a paradox.

Embrace the Paradox

In order to accomplish these two goals in the realm of finances, we put Jody and Taylor's fixed and recurring expenses on autopilot, and we also set up a weekly rhythm in which the ordinary expenses of living were subject to ritualized attention through a family meeting. In the rest of this chapter, you'll learn how to put these two important changes into effect.

And as you set up and maintain your new tools, remember to include some mad money in the budget to allow for a sense of freedom with discretion, as I helped Taylor and Jody to do. Jody would still be able to get out from time to time and order carryout once a week, and Taylor would be able to have lunch with the guys at the greasy spoon, but each would have to choose carefully when to exercise this discretion because the mad money would be finite. Money is all about choices, about taking full responsibility for making active, intentional choices within predetermined limits.

These changes noticeably reduced the sense of chaos and stress in Taylor and Jody's lives—defusing issues that were sparking fights, saving them money, and bringing back a (relative) sense of ease and spontaneity. Whether your baby has already arrived or is soon to come home, similar changes in your own relationship around money can give you the same peace of mind.

Make Intangible Contributions Tangible

Some couples are able to value each person's contributions equally without translating the intangibles into monetary equivalences; others are not. Even gay couples have to struggle through power differentials and perceived inequities to find ways to value the homemaker role (Gianino 2008; Burns, Burgoyne, and Clarke 2008). Taylor and Jody resolved the problem of valuing Jody's contribution by treating the household as a small business. They automated all their fixed expenses, they created a system for managing the ordinary variable expenses, and they each drew a "salary" or allowance in the form of mad money that they didn't have to account to one another for. They held weekly "board meetings" and shared decision making.

I help many couples to value work differently, just as I did with Taylor and Jody. I've even created a spreadsheet of the many tasks that the homemaker does, and I may ask a couple to investigate the real market value of these various functions. (An example of this spreadsheet is available at the end of this chapter.) I put this effort into helping clarify these issues because I've so often seen the issue of money disrupt relationships. There is a profound emotional and psychological dimension to money: it symbolizes what our culture most values and is the agreed-upon currency of worth (Madanes and Madanes 1994). For Taylor and Jody, the increased organization and Jody's newfound sense of being valued and appreciated noticeably decreased the amount of fighting between the couple and created a greater sense of ease within their financial life.

Budgets

Before we could set up a system that would work for them, Taylor and Jody had to tackle their books. This meant identifying their fixed and recurring expenses in great detail. *Fixed expenses* are those that remain the same from month to month: rent or mortgage payments, prorated insurance bills, and so on. Fixed expenses are usually also recurring. *Recurring expenses* are those that keep coming back time and again: gas, water, electricity, auto insurance, and so on. Recurring expenses can be either fixed (always the same and therefore predictable) or variable (fluctuating over the course of time). The mortgage is a good example of an expense that is both fixed (the payment is always the same) and recurring (it's due every month). The water bill may be an example of an expense that is recurring (each month, you get a water bill) but might not be fixed (each month, it changes). The winter-holiday spending is another example of a recurring, varying expense. They come every year, and yet these expenses so often seem to come as a surprise, resulting in budgetary overruns and financial chaos that spill over into the new year. Taylor and Jody each made a list of everything they could think of and then compared notes. For a month they kept track of all their bills to make sure that they hadn't forgotten anything.

Table 7.1 is a rough outline of a format you might use:

Table 7.1: Expenses by Category

Expenses	Fixed	Recurring	Discretionary
Personal			
Business			

Table 7.2 shows a partial list of Taylor and Jody's fixed and recurring expenses (rounded up and with discretionary items below) across several months. You can create a spreadsheet to manage your own.

Table 7.2: Jody and Taylor's Expenses by Category

	January	February	March	April	May
Mortgage/rent	$1985	$1985	$1985	$1985	$1985
Gas/heat	$87	$87	$87	$87	$87
Electricity	$95	$95	$95	$95	$95
Water	$49	$56	$64	$73	$78
Car payment	$448	$448	$448	$448	$448
Auto insurance	$93	$93	$93	$93	$93
Telephone	$109	$110	$107	$112	$109
Cable/Internet	$57	$57	$57	$57	$57
Total	$2923	$2931	$2936	$2950	$2952

Automate Your Accounts

The account that will be used to pay all the fixed and recurring expenses will be automated. We'll call this the household expenses account. Don't use this account for anything else! The important point is to insulate this household checking account from any tendency to view the balance as liquid in any way. So do not set up any checks or debit cards for this account. The ultimate goal is to automate all of this account's transactions, using either automatic draft or recurring electronic check. An automatic draft is one where you give the company you owe permission to draft your account whenever your bill comes due. The drawbacks of this solution are that payment is not under your control, and automatic drafts can be difficult to stop (for instance, if the company you owe makes a mistake and overcharges you). A *recurring electronic check* is another way to automatically pay bills. You can set up this system with your bank, and it lets you retain control over when and whether the payment goes out, decide whether a payment should be stopped (say, if you get into a dispute with the company you owe about a bill), and monitor payments online.

Make use of *equalized payment plans.* Many utility companies will allow you to sign up for an equalized payment plan where they prorate your estimated expenses over a year and then re-evaluate and adjust annually. This allows gas and electricity expenses to be spread out over twelve months so as to absorb the shock of seasonal spikes due to increased usage in hot or cold weather. Put as many accounts as you can into a recurrent plan, as this will transform these regular expenses into fixed, predictable ones, thereby minimizing surprises. Many utilities offer an equalized payment plan as a free service. In my area, for example, both the power company and the gas company offer this service. This means that I pay the same amount year-round so that my electric bill isn't higher in the summer and the gas bill higher in the winter. These utilities typically evaluate your usage patterns and recalibrate your payments once a year, applying any credits and adjusting your rate for the coming year. The year after I replaced my windows, both my electricity and my gas payments went down significantly.

Constrain Variable Expenses

Once you have identified fixed and recurring expenses, once you've automated, and once you've structured as many fixed expenses as possible into equal, predictable, fixed payments, then it's time to count up the variable expenses. Select the variable expenses that recur with some frequency, and begin to tame them with the following four steps.

Calculate the average. Add up each recurring expense for the past year; then, divide it by twelve to obtain a reasonable estimate of the monthly toll it exacts. Let's say that the water bill is one of these recurring but highly variable expenses, ranging from $30 to $78 per month (few people realize that the water company raises the rates during the summer months, precisely when people are using more water to nourish their lawns and fill their swimming pools). If we add all the water bills for the past year and then divide by twelve, we come up with an average figure. According to my local water company, the average for a family of four in my area is $65 per month. Refer back to Table 7.2 here: so far Taylor and Jody's monthly fixed expenses averaged $3,000. But there are a couple of other categories to consider, so this was not the full monthly total that they needed to put into their household account in order to keep this system running smoothly.

Convert irregular payments into fixed line items. Some of your recurring expenses will be ones that occur not on a monthly basis but on some other schedule. Taylor and Jody's automobile insurance is an example of this: it came due twice a year. They divided their total insurance fee by twelve and put that fixed monthly amount into the household account. That way, when the biyearly draft occurred, the money is there waiting and the bill comes as no surprise. (Some companies offer a discount if you pay the year in advance while charging extra for equalizing the payments for you. Therefore, it pays to do the work of stabilizing your payment schedule yourself.) The same principle applies to seasonal-holiday expenses and to vacations. The holidays recur every year, yet many people seem to be surprised when their budget fails and they have to turn to credit cards. Because I am guilty of this, I have opened a special Christmas account at my local credit union. It drafts a fixed amount every month from my checking account, and at the end of October the full savings, plus interest, is moved to my checking account just in time to get a jump on shopping before the malls become totally crazed. I informally do the same with vacations, planning ahead and regularly squirreling away snippets of cash for special travel.

Automate payments to savings, retirement, and health-care savings accounts. Most couples I know overlook these important domains. Taylor's retirement and the family health insurance premiums were already deducted from his salary, so there was no need to take out any more for those expenses. But there was a need to set money aside for emergencies. Something inevitably happens to upset a budget: auto repairs, unexpected medical bills, home repairs, and the list goes on. It's important to plan as much as possible for such future events so that they don't swamp the family budget. By setting aside even a small amount for the roof that will not need to be replaced for another ten years or the medical co-pays that will likely come up this year, you both restrain spending and calm anxiety.

Add up all fixed and recurring monthly expenses. Taylor and Jody's total monthly household expenses were about $3,500 per month (rounded up). This is how much they needed to deposit into the household expenses account so that the balance would always remain sufficient to cover the monthly withdrawals. Ideally, they would put in a little extra so that they have at least one (and preferably several) months' worth of expenses in this account at all times.

Calculate Equitable Contributions

The next challenge is to determine the share of the deposit that each spouse will contribute, making their contributions fair and equitable.

Single-Earner Families

This step was relatively easy for Jody and Taylor because Taylor was the only one with a salary after Miles was born. They lived in North Carolina, where it is assumed that one half of each spouse's salary belongs to the other, so Jody was entitled to fully one half of Taylor's salary to cover her contribution to running the household. This came as something of a shock to Taylor, who justified some of his indulgences with the line that he was the one making money so the money, psychologically speaking, was his to dispense with. Many couples come in to see me all tangled up in resentment and mutual accusations because each one has a different perception of fairness. This is why it's so important to adjust your valuations of each person's work, so each can feel appreciated for what they contribute. (We'll be working more closely on this in the exercises for this chapter.)

Dual-Income Households

When working with dual-income households I usually add up the two figures to come up with a net sum, which is the combined income of the family. I then divide each spouse's income by the combined income to come up with a proportional contribution for each. For easy math, we will assume that the combined income is $100,000. If one spouse's income is $70,000 and the other makes $30,000, then spouse A should contribute 70 percent of the household account and spouse B should contribute 30 percent. Thus, if the total amount that must go into the household account should be $3,000 per month in order to cover all fixed and recurring expenses, then the spouse who makes 70 percent of the income needs to contribute $2,100 every month, and the spouse who makes 30 percent should contribute $900. Although they each have differing amounts to work with, their contributions are proportional and their money is allocated to different budgetary items in an orderly fashion so that each knows what to expect and what their spending limits should be. Of course, for couples who have combined all their finances and accounts without any friction, this step will be unnecessary. But all too often I find that couples combine their funds into one account but keep separate mental accounts. The friction comes when the higher earner wants to hold more power in decision making as a result of earning more. Another pattern that invites trouble happens when a couple combines their funds but divides the bills, again leaving room for the perception of unfairness (usually on the part of the lower earner, but not always). When the accounts are separated not according to each person but into household and discretionary categories (including mad money for each), the arguments necessarily cease or shift. Typically they cease. But sometimes the arguments just shift, exposing hidden resentments that were conveniently masked, hidden by the smoke screen created by the fact that the funds were intermingled.

Sealing the Deal

When Taylor and Jody had set up their system for recurring expenses, they needed to protect and maintain it. This involved a number of actions that helped make the system easier and more automatic. One of these was to use two banks for their accounts. One bank kept their household checking, savings, and HSA (health-care savings account). A second bank kept their variable expenses account. By keeping these accounts hermetically sealed and *irrevocably separate* from one another, they avoided borrowing from Peter to pay Paul and were much more aware of their actual spending habits. Remember, this is just how Taylor and Jody worked things. Other couples will need to have a separate bank for a home-based business, some will keep individual accounts in each spouse's name, and still others will opt to "go green" with the envelope method that I'll explain a little later in this chapter.

Another important way that Jody and Taylor moved to maintain their new system was to reach an understanding about how to use it. A crucial aspect of this understanding was to agree that once their household account was seeded (a full month's worth of expenses was available in advance) and the bills placed on some form of automatic payment, neither one would raid this account for *any* reason, regardless of whether the reasons might feel urgent or even constitute a real emergency. This was an important ingredient to their success: many other couples set up a functional system only to have it fail when they encounter an unexpected situation or money illusions get the best of them, causing them to justify raiding the household account or savings instead of searching for some other solution to the immediate problem. Whole departments at business schools and entire academic journals are dedicated to research on how to create the illusions that will cause you to buy more, so beware and be wise.

Taylor and Jody also started to look at their home finances as a sort of business, which further helped them protect their system. When you run home finances with the same level of professionalism and accountability you bring to the workplace, you can prevent perceptions and emotions from running amok and derailing the long-term partnering objectives of marriage. I encourage all of my couples to hold weekly or biweekly business meetings to go over their finances and any other practical concerns that require problem solving together. This habit frees them to keep their conversations light, fun, and most of all, *positive* (more about weekly meetings a little later). By the time Jody and Taylor implemented these changes, a noticeable sense of ease had taken over their financial lives—with measurable effects on their relationship and their time for Miles. What had once been a bramble was now a neatly ordered garden.

Ritualizing Discretionary Expenses

Once you take care of the basic expenses of living by placing them into a fair, equitable, and automated structure, it is then possible to begin to corral the demon of discretionary expenses. Discretionary expenses are all those that easily slip through one's fingers: groceries, dry cleaning, automobile gas and maintenance, makeup, clothing, eating out, hobbies, and entertainment. Some, like groceries, are necessary; but the amount you spend on these items can vary and usually depends on your tastes. Discretionary expenses can easily upset a carefully crafted budget if you don't take care. When you identify and structure the amount of money available for these expenses, you will be much less likely to use credit cards as income extenders (a common form of denial that gets so many modern Americans in trouble with consumer debt). Before their financial revamp, Jody and Taylor had been trying to keep track of their expenses by putting all the little incidentals on a credit card. The idea was to simplify record keeping and pay off the card every month, but this had only gotten them into trouble. By the time they had consolidated their debts twice, they didn't need much persuasion to realize that this smoke-and-mirrors system wasn't really working for them all that well. In fact, research shows that people spend on average 34 percent to 64 percent more when they use either plastic or checks because there is simply not the same sense of limitation with checks and credit cards that there is with cash—the illusion is just that powerful (Prelec and Loewenstein 1998; Prelec and Simester 2001; Srivastava and Raghubir 2002). Transitioning over to a cash system involves considerable effort and self-discipline. However, even though any system tends to be slippery in today's complex world, the effort pays off in spades over a lifetime.

In order for this cash system to work well, you will need to monitor the discretionary expenses account more closely—hence the need for a ritual. The number and variety of methods that people devise for managing this category of expenses is rich and varied. The bottom line is to use whatever works best for you. I like Sarah Ban Breathnach's recommendation from her book *Simple Abundance* (Ban Breathnach 1995): set a regular time and place for monitoring these expenses and making the ritual as pleasant as possible. Here's her entry for October 25:

> Once, in a flush season when I had no reason to worry about money, I created a ritual for paying bills. At the beginning and the middle of each month, I would set aside a half hour to quietly, consciously settle my accounts. I'd clear my desktop, leaving only my bills, checkbook, calculator, envelopes, and stamps in view. As I worked, I'd play soft, soothing music, and sip a lovely cup of tea, and pay loving attention to what I was doing. As a result, I actually began to enjoy the experience. When leaner times arrived, I still relied on the power of ritual to keep me positive. If I was feeling frightened, I would retrieve the memories of when I paid bills with ease, recalling the positive feeling of plenty: well-being, peace, security, freedom. Since our subconscious minds cannot distinguish between reality and fantasy, I would begin to relax. Even if my reality was not set during a season of plenty, I gradually came to know contentment in the season of enough.

Envelopes or Checking?

Many of my clients have opted to use the "envelope method" for managing the discretionary expense account rather than using a checking account. They find that this system helps make the limits of their finances more palpable and real for them. The *envelope method* involves literally putting the cash for each of the line items in your discretionary budget into an envelope labeled for that category. You can then borrow from one category for an expense in another, but the finitude of the cash being shifted around remains tangible and protects against money illusions. This way you take the cash from the envelope marked "Groceries" to pay for food, cash from the envelope marked "Gas" to put fuel in the car, cash from the envelope marked "Entertainment" to go to the movies, and so on. When the cash is out, your make do until the next time you get paid. If you have to borrow from the entertainment envelope to put fuel in the car, leaving very little left for entertainment, then maybe you will need to play cards on Saturday instead of renting a movie. When forced to face reality in this way, many people become very conscious and very creative about ways to save money and ways to have fun on the cheap (Prelec and Loewenstein 1998; Soman 2003).

If you opt to use a checking account for your discretionary expenses, I recommend that you keep the check register electronically using something like Microsoft Money or Quicken, and that you reconcile the account *weekly*. If you are so lucky as to have more income than expenses by a wide margin and more disposable income than you know what to do with, then this rigorous check-in process might be optional for you. Others will probably benefit from setting a weekly ritual of time, place, and ambiance. Jody did a one-time decluttering of her home desk, she developed a filing system so that everything would be organized and available when tax time rolled around, and she used a pretty hat box that she found at a garage sale to keep her current bills in. Then she programmed a specific playlist into her iPod. Now, every Sunday afternoon at four o'clock, when she is well rested and preparing to meet the upcoming week, she sits down with a cup of hot herbal tea to pay bills and reconcile the checkbook.

Giving the Devil His Due

It's not enough to automate fixed and recurring expenses and subject all discretionary expenses to a pleasing and chaos-containing ritual. There must somehow be some small amount of money in the budget that you don't have to be accountable for: mad money. From your discretionary expense account, pay yourself and your partner a weekly cash allowance that you are free to play with as you wish without having to render accounting to the other partner. This allows each to feel some measure of independence and to indulge the "wild side" without threatening the larger family financial system.

I use my mad money for tango, lunches out, and Starbucks. If I overindulge in lunch on the run, I might have to miss a Saturday night of dancing cheek to cheek, so I'm motivated to keep my intake of caffeine and processed foods in check. My physical, financial, and emotional health has benefited in more than one way as a result. I work with my patients in identifying their particular behavioral goals and weaknesses so that we can use the mad-money category to greatest advantage. With this small fund, we can create behavioral contingencies that maximize pleasure and behavioral control. Taylor and Jody noticed an interesting trend in their mad money over the first several months of using this method. Taylor went from being a junk-food junkie to bringing home fresh flowers once a week or so. When spring came, they rediscovered their joy in gardening and started raising some vegetables of their own. They even joined a vintage dance group and took the baby to class strapped in his baby backpack. These are things they never would have done had they still been so stressed-out about money. Getting on top of finances is one of the fastest ways you can destress your life and find more quality time as a family.

Here's a table showing data for the first five months that Taylor and Jody sorted out their discretionary expenses:

Table 7.3: Taylor and Jody's Discretionary Spending

	January	February	March	April	May
Groceries	$650	$650	$722	$737	$668
Netflix	$24	$24	$24	$24	$24
Auto gas	$347	$350	$379	$385	$383
Dry Cleaning	$37	$32	$28	$38	$18
Entertainment	$143	$84	$54	$99	$109
Eating out	$250	$311	$170	$140	$155
Diaper service	$72	$72	$72	$80	$80
Babysitters	$200	$280	$105	$220	$250
Savings	$101	$150	$0	$78	$0
Makeup	$51	$0	$19	$0	$22
Toiletries	$38	$41	$44	$56	$43
Clothing	$104	$23	$200	$600	$600
Mad $$	$400	$400	$600		

Notice that in March and May they had no savings, and in April they only put $78 into savings. Rather than go into debt that they would have to pay off later, Taylor and Jody opted to use the savings account as the catchall for budget overruns. This was a natural extension of their commitment to a cash economy with regard to their variable and discretionary expenses. Notice too that they found a mere $50 each per week in mad money to be too tight, so they raised their allowances in March to $70 per week, which they found more comfortable. Truth be told, some of the mad money went to extend the eating out category, but since it was discretionary cash that didn't have to be accounted for under this system, they treated one another. After looking over their expenses for the five-month trial period, they agreed to make some cuts in regular expenses and try to save more. Knowing that their penny-pinching had a purpose helped them to meet this goal by year's end. Naturally, their increased sense of control around money not only helped them save more (itself a stress-reducing result) but also gave them more time and mental attention to devote to each other and to Miles.

Running the Household Like a Business

When Jody finished paying bills and reconciling the checkbook, she and Taylor had their family "board meeting." They found that Miles would tolerate his swing just long enough and sometimes they even managed to tuck the meeting in during one of his naps. Although naps are growing more infrequent these days, Jody and Taylor discovered that Miles could learn to wait—teaching him to do so was harder on them than on him.

During their mini-meetings, Jody kept Taylor up to date on the family budget and they updated one another about how they were doing with their cash expenses. These meetings turned out to be an eye-opener for Taylor, who used to be the one complaining about Jody's spending. When he had to account for his own outlays, it turned out that Taylor's drive-through indiscretions added up to raids on the eating-out line item. It was his stops at Starbucks on the way to work and his lunch expenses that largely drove their reassessment of the mad money category. Jody sometimes used her mad money to extend the babysitter budget, too, which illustrates that the system is a framework with some room for flexibility—but not a lot. During their board meetings, Jody and Taylor would problem solve and plan around any unforeseen spending or "business"-related decisions. Jody didn't like feeling like she was "reporting to" Taylor at first, but after a couple of months she realized that the little extra effort paid huge dividends in mutual respect—especially once Taylor was found with egg on his face and she had a chance to be gracious. Not only did Taylor respect her work as the person managing their household finances, Jody respected herself more for her contributions. And when they finish the meeting each Sunday, they cook dinner together and play with the baby, reminding themselves that the best things in life are free.

Jody and Taylor took to this system like fish to water. Taylor felt confident that even though Jody was not generating income in the same sense as his salary, her contributions were real and tangible; Jody felt free to once again exercise her autonomy and competence. Taylor returned to being the fun-loving guy Jody fell in love with; Jody, the sophisticated woman Taylor chose for his life partner. They felt much more in control of their finances, their spending was no longer mood dependent, and they didn't bicker about who was getting over on the other. They were also becoming wiser spenders. The grocery bill went up in the spring because they were buying fresh fruit, vegetables, and organic meats at the farmer's market, but their entertainment and eating-out expenses went down. Their savings also increased. As they looked over their spreadsheets for the past several months, they came to appreciate the rewards of the effort they had put into the difficult task of changing their behavior and breaking free from illusions about money.

Money and Happiness

Countless books have been written on the topic of money and happiness. While it is true that poverty, not having enough to meet the basic necessities of life, puts people at risk for all sorts of ills, it's not true that having more will necessarily make you happier. It seems that people base their happiness at least in part on their aspirations, and, as they attain more success or prosperity, their aspirations increase accordingly (Easterlin 2001). Thus, the level of happiness in the United States has decreased since 1950, presumably because we Americans have continued to raise the level of our aspirations to match our increasing prosperity. Also, our mass media tend to portray opulence as the norm, setting our expectations to unattainable, over-the-rainbow standards. But prosperity and aspirations have remained largely unchanged in other countries. In one study comparing the happiness of Americans to Brits since the 1950s, the researchers found that "[r]eported levels of well-being have declined over the last quarter of a century in the US; life satisfaction has run approximately flat through time in Britain" (Blanchflower and Oswald 2004, 1359).

According to Harvard psychologist Daniel Gilbert, the keys to happiness are in our ability to manufacture "synthetic happiness," the kind of happiness that comes from the habits of thought that we develop throughout life for absorbing disappointments, rejection, failure, discomfort, and tragedy (2005b). According to a talk he gave at TEDGlobal 2005, the keys to happiness are mostly in the things that money cannot buy, and for what remains, habits of thought can be learned and cultivated (2005a). The habits of thought that protect from depression and generate synthetic happiness are taught in families, social groups, and cultures or learned with a qualified professional in therapy. You can develop the habits of thought that will manufacture the brain chemicals and, over time, will make the dendritic connections in your brain involved in happiness so you, too, can enjoy the most amazing season of your life—early parenthood, when your kids are still little.

Exercises for Chapter 7

Exercise 1: Valuing Intangible Contributions

Get on the Internet and find out the costs for each of the services in the lists that follow. Create a spreadsheet listing the estimates you have obtained in each area.

Note: *Services not included must go into a separate line item and one to three estimates should be obtained for those services.*

Housework

As you troll for information about the prices of housekeeping services, identify what exactly is provided for the price. This may include (or exclude) items like: vacuuming, heavy cleaning of the kitchen, making beds, changing bed linens, scrubbing the bathtub and toilets, sanitizing mold from shower doors, dusting, wiping down walls, cleaning mirrors and windows, picking up toys, organizing closets, putting away out-of-season clothes, organizing drawers, loading and unloading the dishwasher, putting dishes away, putting laundry away, and handwashing heavily soiled pots and pans.

- **Cleaning Services**: When I Googled "cleaning services" for my area, I got several different listings. Each indicated that their prices depended on certain variables. It would be possible to create a spreadsheet and compare prices and services with a few phone calls.

- **Laundry**: Some dry cleaners offer pickup and delivery service, and some offer wash, dry, and fold services. Many of my clients have had good luck placing an ad in the local student newspaper, interviewing, and getting references. They were able to find someone to clean, do laundry, and pick up the groceries and dry cleaning for a flat hourly rate.

- **Grocery Pickup**: Many of my clients have discovered the convenience of shopping for groceries online (but this service isn't offered everywhere). You could shop online at home while the baby is napping. Or, some parents find it convenient for one to order the groceries online or by phone and the other parent to pick it up.

Organizing Services

- **Home Office**: This category can include organizing the desk, the filing system, and receipts and finances. Professional organizing services are listed online, and there is even a National Association of Professional Organizers (NAPO) that certifies professional organizers.

- **Bookkeeping**: Just balancing the checkbook, paying the bills, and filing the appropriate records for tax time is a job in itself. Bookkeeping can include entering and paying bills, checking for duplicates, calling merchants who have overcharged, stopping unnecessary services, and so on. To find out what it's worth to you, search for "bookkeepers" in your area.

- **Tax Preparation:** It takes time to enter financial information into TurboTax and do it yourself, and even then you have to be sufficiently organized to have all the necessary information available to you when the time comes. But if you outsource tax preparation, that costs too—so go ahead and look it up. Find out what this contribution is worth in monetary terms.

Child Care

◆ **Postpartum Doula:** Many of my clients benefit from hiring a postpartum doula to help them get adjusted to the role of parenting a newborn. To find out how much this service is worth, check out DONA International (Doulas of North America) online.

◆ **Day Care:** If you or your spouse has to take off work to take care of the kid(s), what is the cost in monetary terms? What will it cost you to replace that help with some other kind of child care like a drop-in center or a sitter? Find at least three different types of child care and price them.

◆ **Nanny Services:** For those couples who decide that it's best or easiest for one to stay home with baby for a few years, pricing au pairs and nanny services can help bring home the value of full-time child care.

Nutrition

◆ **Feeding the Family:** This is a big one and includes meal planning, grocery shopping, and food preparation. The area where I live has recently experienced a proliferation of personal chef services—people who will take all the thinking, shopping, and cooking out of your life for the entire week. Just what does this kind of household contribution cost to replace? Find out for yourself.

Yard Care

- **Establishing Care**: This includes getting a garden going—planning the landscaping, shopping for plants, preparing the soil, and planting.

- **Maintenance**: What does it take to keep the garden or yard looking good (or at least alive)? This category includes mowing, edging, weeding, picking produce, feeding, and insect control.

Following is an example of the spreadsheet some clients use to organize their expenses. Feel free to create one like it for your family.

Figure 7.1: Valuing Homecare Spreadsheet Example

	Estimate 1	Estimate 2	Estimate 3
Housecleaning services			
Maintenance cleaning & tidying			
Vacuuming and deep cleaning			
Bathrooms & mopping			
Meal preparation			
Menu planning			
Grocery shopping			
Cooking			
Wash/dry/fold services			
Dry cleaning pickup & delivery			
Personal organizer			
Bookkeeping & bill paying			
Tax preparation			

Child care

Full time/nanny

Emergency/drop-in

Yard care

Mowing, etc.

Seeding & aeration

Fertilizing & pest control

Mulching

Exercise 2: Ritualizing Variable Expenses

Sarah Ban Breathnach created a ritual to help her stay positive while she paid her bills. It came in hTaylor, especially when times were lean or her spirits were low. She kept her bills in an attractive box and used soft music and hot herbal tea to soothe herself while she wrote out her checks (1995).

What kind of ritual will you create? How will you regularize your bill paying and make it pleasant? Do you already have an existing habit that you could link this activity to (like a habit of cleaning house on Saturday morning or folding laundry on Sunday afternoon)? Linking a new behavior to an existing habit is a very helpful way to jump-start new behaviors. And having a reward that is meaningful will also help the new habit take root. What incentives/props/accountability systems do you think you need in order to generate the repetitions necessary to establish this habit?

Steps to take:

- Choose a time of day and a day of the week.

- Set the time apart and make it pleasant (consider pleasing all five of your senses).

- Make the space pleasant.

- Alert others in the household, to protect the time from interruptions.

- Reward yourself afterward.

When you consider your reward, you don't necessarily have to limit yourself to tangible things. While a piece of cTaylor or a cookie might be a great reward, don't forget about those that appeal in other ways. For instance, you can devote a small bit of time to noticing just how good it feels to complete your ritual. You can journal about your success, writing down all the ways that maintaining this ritual helps you and makes you feel better. And then, instead of (or in addition to) these intangible rewards, you can make sure you have a tangible, low-cost reward—preferably something special to you. Maybe bill night could become movie night? What do you think will work for you?

References

Abad, V. C., and C. Guilleminault. 2005. Sleep and psychiatry. *Dialogues in Clinical Neuroscience* 7:291–303.

Abdool, Z., R. Thakar, and A. H. Sultan. 2009. Postpartum female sexual function: A review. *European Journal of Obstetrics & Gynecology and Reproductive Biology*. 145 (2):133-137.

Abramson, L. Y., G. I. Metalsky, and L. B. Alloy. 1989. Hopelessness depression: A theory-based subtype of depression. *Psychological Review* 96 (2):358–372.

Abramson, L. Y., M. E. Seligman, and J. D. Teasdale. 1978. Learned helplessness in humans: Critique and reformulation. *Journal of Abnormal Psychology* 87 (1):49–74.

Ahlborg, T., L. G. Dahlof, and L. R. Hallberg. 2005. Quality of the intimate and sexual relationship in first-time parents six months after delivery. *Journal of Sex Research* 42 (2):167–174.

Ahrold, T. K., and C. M. Meston. 2009. Effects of SNS activation on SSRI-induced sexual side effects differ by SSRI. *Journal of Sex & Marital Therapy* 35 (4):311–319.

Ainsworth, M. D. 1969. Object relations, dependency, and attachment: A theoretical review of the infant-mother relationship. *Child Development* 40 (4):969–1025.

Ainsworth, M. D., and S. M. Bell. 1970. Attachment, exploration, and separation: Illustrated by the behavior of one-year-olds in a strange situation. *Child Development* 41 (1):49–67.

Ainsworth, M. S. 1979. Infant mother attachment. *American Psychologist* 34 (10):932–937.

Ainsworth, M. S., and J. Bowlby. 1991. An ethological approach to personality development. *American Psychologist* 46 (4):333–341.

Alder, E. M. 1989. Sexual behaviour in pregnancy, after childbirth, and during breast-feeding. *Baillieres Clinical Obstetrics and Gynaecology* 3 (4):805–821.

Alexander, C. J. 2001. Developmental attachment and gay and lesbian adoptions. *Journal of Gay & Lesbian Social Services: Issues in Practice, Policy & Research* 13 (3):93–97.

Allen, S. M., and A. J. Hawkins. 1999. Maternal gatekeeping: Mothers' beliefs and behaviors that inhibit greater father involvement in family work. *Journal of Marriage and the Family* 61 (February):199–212.

American Psychiatric Association. 2000. *Diagnostic and Statistical Manual of Mental Disorders.* 4th ed. Text Revision. Washington, DC: American Psychiatric Association.

Andersen, B. L., J. M. Cyranowski, and S. Aarestad. 2000. Beyond artificial, sex-linked distinctions to conceptualize female sexuality: Comment on Baumeister. *Psychological Bulletin* 126 (3):380–384.

Anderson, S. A., and R. M. Sabatelli. 2003. *Family Interaction: A Multigenerational Developmental Perspective.* Boston: Allyn & Bacon.

Ayduk, O., G. Downey, and M. Kim. 2001. Rejection sensitivity and depressive symptoms in women. *Personality and Social Psychology Bulletin* 27 (7):868.

Ayduk, O., R. Mendoza-Denton, W. Mischel, G. Downey, P. K. Peake, and M. Rodriguez. 2000. Regulating the interpersonal self: Strategic self-regulation for coping with rejection sensitivity. *Journal of Personality and Social Psychology* 79 (5):776–792.

Ayduk, O., W. Mischel, and G. Downey. 2002. Attentional mechanisms linking rejection to hostile reactivity: The role of "hot" versus "cool" focus. *Psychological Science* 13 (5):443–449.

Ballard, C., and R. Davies. 1996. Postnatal depression in fathers. *International Review of Psychiatry* 8 (1):65–71.

Ballard, C. G., R. Davis, P. C. Cullen, R. N. Mohan, and C. Dean. 1994. Prevalence of postnatal psychiatric morbidity in mothers and fathers. *British Journal of Psychiatry* 164 (6):782–788.

Ban Breathnach, S. 1995. *Simple Abundance: A Daybook of Comfort and Joy.* New York: Warner Books.

Bandura, A. 2006. Toward a psychology of human agency. *Perspectives on Psychological Science* 1 (2):164–180.

Banks, A. E. 2001. *Post-Traumatic Stress Disorder: Relationships and Brain Chemistry.* Wellesley, MA: Jean Baker Miller Institute.

Barnett, R. C., and J. S. Hyde. 2001. Women, men, work, and family. *American Psychologist* 56 (10):781–796.

Barrett, G., E. Pendry, J. Peacock, C. Victor, R. Thakar, and I. Manyonda. 2000. Women's sexual health after childbirth. *British Journal of Obstetrics and Gynaecology* 107 (2):186–95.

Barrett, L. F., and E. Bliss-Moreau. 2009. She's emotional. He's having a bad day: Attributional explanations for emotion stereotypes. *Emotion* 9 (5):649–658.

Bartlett, E. E. 2004. The effects of fatherhood on the health of men: A review of the literature. *Journal of Men's Health & Gender* 1 (2–3):159–169.

Basson, R. 2001. Using a different model for female sexual response to address women's problematic low sexual desire. *Journal of Sex & Marital Therapy* 27 (5):395–403.

Basson, R. 2002a. A model of women's sexual arousal. *Journal of Sex & Marital Therapy* 28:1–10.

Basson, R. 2002b. Women's sexual desire: Disordered or misunderstood? *Journal of Sex & Marital Therapy* 28 (Suppl1):17–28.

Basson, R. 2003. Biopsychosocial models of women's sexual response: Applications to management of "desire disorders." *Sexual and Relationship Therapy* 18 (1):107–115.

Basson, R., S. Leiblum, L. Brotto, L. Derogatis, J. Fourcroy, K. Fugl-Meyer, et al. 2003. Definitions of women's sexual dysfunction reconsidered : Advocating expansion and revision. *Journal of Psychosomatic Obstetrics and Gynecology* 24 (4):221–229.

Bastiaansen, J. A. J., M. Thioux, and C. Keysers. 2009. Evidence for mirror systems in emotions. *Philosophical Transactions of the Royal Society B: Biological Sciences* 364 (1528):2391–2404.

Baumeister, R. F. 2000. Gender differences in erotic plasticity: The female sex drive as socially flexible and responsive. *Psychological Bulletin* 126 (3):347–374.

Baumeister, R. F., C. N. DeWall, N. J. Ciarocco, and J. M. Twenge. 2005. Social exclusion impairs self-regulation. *Journal of Personality and Social Psychology* 88 (4):589–604.

Baumeister, R. F., and M. R. Leary. 1995. The need to belong: Desire for interpersonal attachments as a fundamental human motivation. *Psychological Bulletin* 117 (3):497–529.

Baumeister, R. F., J. M. Twenge, and C. K. Nuss. 2002. Effects of social exclusion on cognitive processes: Anticipated aloneness reduces intelligent thought. *Journal of Personality and Social Psychology* 83 (4):817–827.

Baxter, J., B. Hewitt, and M. Haynes. 2008. Life course transitions and housework: Marriage, parenthood, and time on housework. *Journal of Marriage and Family* 70 (May):259–272.

Beaulieu-Provost, D., C. C. Simard, and A. Zadra. 2009. Making sense of dream experiences: A multidimensional approach to beliefs about dreams. *Dreaming* 19 (3):119–134.

Beauregard, M. 2009. Effect of mind on brain activity: Evidence from neuroimaging studies of psychotherapy and placebo effect. *Nordic Journal of Psychiatry* 63 (1):5–16.

Beck, A. T. 2005. The current state of cognitive therapy. *Archives of General Psychiatry* 62 (9):953–959.

Beck, A. T., and B. A. Alford. 2009. *Depression: Causes and Treatment* (2nd ed.). Baltimore, MD: University of Pennsylvania Press.

Beck, C. T. 1998. The effects of postpartum depression on child development: a meta analysis. *Archives of Psychiatric Nursing* 12:12–20.

Beck, C. T. 2001. Predictors of postpartum depression. *Nursing Research* 50 (5):275–285.

Becker, A. E. 1998. Postpartum illness in Fiji: A sociosomatic perspective. *Psychosomatic Medicine* 60 (4):431–438.

Becker, A. E., and D. T. S. Lee. 2002. Indigenous models for attenuation of postpartum depression: case studies from Fiji and Hong Kong. In *The World Mental Health Casebook*, edited by A. Cohen, A. Kleinman, and B. Saraceno. New York: Kluwer/Academic Publishers.

Begley, S. 2010. The depressing news about antidepressants. *Newsweek Magazine*, January 29.

Belkin, L. 2009. Let the kid be. *New York Times*, May 31. http://www.nytimes.com/2009/05/31/magazine/31wwln-lede-t.html?_r=1&ref=lisa_belkin.

Bell, B. G., and J. Belsky. 2008. Parents, parenting, and children's sleep problems: Exploring reciprocal effects. *British Journal of Developmental Psychology* 26 (4):579–593.

Bell, S. M., and M. S. Ainsworth. 1972. Infant crying and maternal responsiveness. *Child Development* 43:1171–1190.

Belsky, Jay. 1985. Exploring individual differences in marital change across the transition to parenthood: The role of violated expectations. *Journal of Marriage and Family* 47 (4):1037–1044.

Benazon, N. R. 2000. Predicting negative spousal attitudes toward depressed persons: A test of Coyne's Interpersonal Model. *Journal of Abnormal Psychology* 109 (3):550–554.

Benazon, N. R., and J. C. Coyne. 2000. Living with a depressed spouse. *Journal of Family Psychology* 14 (1):71–79.

Berger, M., D. VanCalker, and D. Riemann. 2003. Sleep and manipulations of the sleep-wake rhythm in depression. *Acta Psychiatria Scandanavica* 418:83–91.

Bibring, G. 1959. Some considerations of the psychological processes in pregnancy. *The Psychoanalytic Study of the Child* 14:113–121.

Billiard, M., M. Partinen, T. Roth, and C. Shapiro. 1994. Sleep and psychiatric disorders. *Journal of Psychosomatic Research,* 38 (Supplement 1):1–2.

Blanchflower, D. G., and A. J. Oswald. 2004. Well-being over time in Britain and the USA. *Journal of Public Economics* 88:1359–1386.

Bloch, M., R. C. Daly, and D. R. Rubinow. 2003. Endocrine factors in the etiology of postpartum depression. *Comprehensive Psychiatry* 44 (3):234–246.

Bloch, M., P. Schmidt, M. Danaceau, J. Murphy, L. Nieman, and D. Rubinow. 2000. Effects of gonadal steroids in women with a history of postpartum depression. *American Journal of Psychiatry* 157:924–930.

Blood, A. J., and R. J. Zatorre. 2001. Intensely pleasurable responses to music correlate with activity in brain regions implicated in reward and emotion. *Proceedings of the National Academy of Sciences of the United States of America* 98 (20):11818–11823.

Blyton, D. M., C. E. Sullivan, and N. J. Edwards. 2002. Lactation is associated with an increase in slow-wave sleep in women. *Sleep Research* 11:297–303.

Boren, J. J., A. M. Leventhal, and H. E. Pigott. 2009. Just how effective are antidepressant medications? Results of a major new study. *Journal of Contemporary Psychotherapy* 39 (2):93–100.

Bosch, J. A., E. J. C. de Geus, E. C. I. Veerman, J. Hoogstraten, and A. V. Nieuw Amerongen. 2003. Innate secretory immunity in response to laboratory stressors that evoke distinct patterns of cardiac autonomic activity. *Psychosomatic Medicine* 65 (2):245–258.

Bosch, J. A., M. Turkenburg, K. Nazmi, E. C. I. Veerman, E. J. C. de Geus, and A. V. Nieuw Amerongen. 2003. Stress as a determinant of saliva-mediated adherence and coadherence of oral and non-oral microorganisms. *Psychosomatic Medicine* 65 (4):604–612.

Bost, K. K., M. J. Cox, M. R. Burchinal, and C. Payne. 2002. Structural and supportive changes in couples' family and friendship networks across the transition to parenthood. *Journal of Marriage and Family* 64 (2):517–531.

Boyington, J., A. Johnson, and L. Carter-Edwards. 2007. Dissatisfaction with body size among low-income, postpartum Black women. *Journal of Obstetric, Gynecologic, & Neonatal Nursing: Clinical Scholarship for the Care of Women, Childbearing Families, & Newborns* 36 (2):144–151.

Bradford, A., and C. M. Meston. 2006. The impact of anxiety on sexual arousal in women. *Behaviour Research and Therapy* 44:1067–1077.

Bradford, A., and C. M. Meston. 2009. Placebo response in the treatment of women's sexual dysfunctions: A review and commentary. *Journal of Sex & Marital Therapy* 35 (3):164–181.

Brady, J. V. 1958. Ulcers in "executive" monkeys. *Scientific American* 199 (3):95–104.

Braun, S. 2006. Gay and lesbian adoptive parenting. American Psychological Association 2006 Convention Presentation.

Brennan, A., S. Marshall-Lucette, S. Ayers, and H. Ahmed. 2007. A qualitative exploration of the Couvade syndrome in expectant fathers. *Journal of Reproductive and Infant Psychology* 25 (1):18–39.

Bretherton, I. 1992. The origins of attachment theory: John Bowlby and Mary Ainsworth. *Developmental Psychology* 28 (5):759–775.

Brinker, J. K., and D. J. Dozois. 2009. Ruminative thought style and depressed mood. *Journal of Clinical Psychology* 65 (Jan):1–19.

Brotto, L. A., R. Basson, and M. Luria. 2008. A mindfulness-based group psychoeducational intervention targeting sexual arousal disorder in women. *Journal of Sexual Medicine* 5 (7):1646–1659.

Brotto, L. A., R. Basson, and J. S. T. Woo. 2009. Female sexual arousal disorders. In *Clinical Manual of Sexual Disorders*, edited by R. Balon and R. T. Segraves. Arlington, VA: American Psychiatric Publishing, Inc.

Brown, K. W., and R. M. Ryan. 2003. The benefits of being present: Mindfulness and its role in psychological well-being. *Journal of Personality and Social Psychology* 84 (4):822–848.

Bucove, A. 1964. Postpartum psychoses in the male. *Bulletin of the New York Academy of Medicine* 40:961–971.

Burns, A. B., J. S. Brown, E. A. Plant, N. Sachs-Ericsson, and T. E. Joiner Jr. 2006. On the specific depressotypic nature of excessive reassurance-seeking. *Personality and Individual Differences* 40 (1):135–145.

Burns, D., and S. Nolen-Hoeksema. 1991. Coping styles, homework compliance, and the effectiveness of cognitive-behavioral therapy. *Journal of Consulting and Clinical Psychology* 59 (305–311).

Burns, M., C. Burgoyne, and V. Clarke. 2008. Financial affairs? Money management in same-sex relationships. *The Journal of Socio-Economics* 37 (2):481–501.

Byrne, R. 2007. *The Secret.* New York: Atria Publishing.

Carro, M. G., K. E. Grant, I. H. Gotlib, and B. E. Compas. 1993. Postpartum depression and child development: An investigation of mothers and fathers as sources of risk and resilience. *Development and Psychopathology* 5 (4):567–579.

Cash, T. F. 1997. *The Body Image Workbook: An 8-Step Program for Learning to Like Your Looks.* Oakland, CA: New Harbinger Publications.

Cash, T. F., C. L. Maikkula, and M. S. Yamamiya. 2004. Baring the body in the bedroom: body image, sexual self-schemas, and sexual functioning among college women and men. *Electronic Journal of Human Sexuality* 7.

Caspi, A. 2000. The child is father of the man: Personality continuities from childhood to adulthood. *Journal of Personality and Social Psychology* 78 (1):158–172.

Caspi, A., D. J. Bem, and G. H. Elder Jr. 1989. Continuities and consequences of interactional styles across the life course. *Journal of Personality* 57 (2):375–406.

Caspi, A., and T. E. Moffitt. 1991. Individual differences are accentuated during periods of social change: The sample case of girls at puberty. *Journal of Personality and Social Psychology* 61 (1):157–168.

Ciesla, J. A., and J. E. Roberts. 2007. Rumination, negative cognition, and their interactive effects on depressed mood. *Emotion* 7 (3):555–565.

Chaudron, L. 2003. Is postpartum psychosis a bipolar variant? A phenomenological question. *Psychiatric Times* 20 (7):54.

Chen, S., T. English, and K. Peng. 2006. Self-verification and contextualized self-views. *Society for Personality and Social Psychology* 32 (7):930–942.

Christakis, N. A., and F. Fowler. 2007. The spread of obesity in a large social network over 32 years. *New England Journal of Medicine* 357 (4):370–379.

Christakis, N. A., and J. H. Fowler. 2008. The collective dynamics of smoking in a large social network. *New England Journal of Medicine* 358 (21):2249–2258.

Clark, A., H. Skouteris, E. H. Wertheim, S. J. Paxton, and J. Milgrom. 2009. The relationship between depression and body dissatisfaction across pregnancy and the postpartum: A prospective study. *Journal of Health Psychology* 14 (1):27–35.

Clark-Flory, T. 2009. Why do women have sex? *Salon.com*. October 5. http://www .salon.com/life/feature/2009/10/05/why_women_have_sex.

Clinton, J. F. 1986. Expectant fathers at risk for couvade. *Nursing Research* 35 (5):290–295.

Cohan, C. L., and S. Kleinbaum. 2002. Toward a greater understanding of the cohabitation effect: Premarital cohabitation and marital communication. *Journal of Marriage and Family* 64:180–192.

Cohelo, R. 1949. The significance of the Couvade among the Black Caribs. *Man* 49:51–53.

Collier, R. 2009. Recession stresses mental health system. *Canadian Medical Association Journal* 181 (3–4):e48–e49.

Conner, G. K., and V. Denson. 1990. Expectant fathers' response to pregnancy: Review of literature and implications for research in high-risk pregnancy. *Journal of Perinatal and Neonatal Nursing* 4 (2):33–42.

Coontz, S. 1992. *The Way We Never Were: American Families and the Nostalgia Trap*. New York: Basic Books.

Costner, H. L. *The Changing Folkways of Parenthood: A Content Analysis*. Manchester, NH: Ayers Company Publishing.

Covey, S. 1989. *The Seven Habits of Highly Effective People*. New York: Free Press.

Cowan, C. P., and P. Cowan. 1995. Interventions to ease the transition to parenthood: Why they are needed and what they can do. *Family Relations*, 44 (4):412–423.

Cowan, C. P., P. A. Cowan, G. Heming, E. Garrett, W. S. Coysh, H. Curtis-Boles, and A. J. Boles III. 1985. Transitions to parenthood: His, hers, and theirs. *Journal of Family Issues* 6:451–481.

Crenshaw, D. 2008. *The Myth of Multitasking: How "Doing It All" Gets Nothing Done*: San Francisco, CA: Jossey-Bass.

Critchley, H. D. 2009. Psychophysiology of neural, cognitive and affective integration: fMRI and autonomic indicants. *International Journal of Psychophysiology* 73 (2):88–94.

Crowe, M., and S. Luty. 2005. The process of change in interpersonal psychotherapy (IPT) for depression: A case study for the new IPT therapist. *Psychiatry* 68 (1):43–54.

Cutrona, C. E. 1983. Causal attributions and perinatal depression. *Journal of Abnormal Psychology* 92 (2):161–172.

D'Sa, C., and R. S. Duman. 2002. Antidepressants and neuroplasticity. *Bipolar Disorders* 4:183–194.

Davis, S. N., and T. N. Greenstein. 2004. Cross-national variations in the division of household labor. *Journal of Marriage and Family* 66 (5):1260–1271.

Deave, T., D. Johnson, and J. Ingram. 2008. Transition to parenthood: The needs of parents in pregnancy and early parenthood. *BMC Pregnancy and Childbirth* 8 (30).

DeLange, F. P., A. Koers, J. S. Kalkman, G. Bleijenberg, P. Hagoort, J. W. M. van der Meer, and I. Toni. 2008. Increase in prefrontal cortical volume following cognitive behavioural therapy in patients with chronic fatigue syndrome. *Brain* 131:2172–2180.

Demo, D. H., and A. C. Acock. 1993. Family diversity and the division of domestic labor: How much have things really changed? *Family Relations* 42 (3):323–331.

Demo, D. H., and M. J. Cox. 2000. Families with young children: A review of research in the 1990s. *Journal of Marriage and the Family* 62 (4):876–895.

Dennis, C.-L., and L. Ross. 2006. Women's perceptions of partner support and conflict in the development of postpartum depressive symptoms. *Journal of Advanced Nursing* 56 (6):588–599.

DeRaedt, R. 2006. Does neuroscience hold promise for the further development of behavior therapy? The case of emotional change after exposure in anxiety and depression. *Scandinavian Journal of Psychology* 47:225–236.

Derryberry, D., and M. K. Rothbart. 1988. Arousal, affect, and attention as components of temperament. *Journal of Personality and Social Psychology* 55 (6):958–966.

DeRubeis, R. J., L. A. Gelfand, T. Z. Tang, and A. D. Simons. 1999. Medications versus cognitive behavior therapy for severely depressed outpatients: Mega-analysis of four randomized comparisons. *American Journal of Psychiatry* 156:1007–1013.

DeRubeis, R. J., S. D. Hollon, J. D. Amsterdam, R. C. Shelton, P. R. Young, R. M. Salomon, et al. 2005. Cognitive therapy vs medications in the treatment of moderate to severe depression. *Archives of General Psychiatry* 62 (4):409–416.

Dhand, R., and H. Sohal. 2006. Good sleep, bad sleep! The role of daytime naps in healthy adults. *Current Opinion in Pulmonary Medicine* 12 (6):379–382.

Diego, M. A., T. Field, M. Hernandez-Reif, C. Cullen, S. Schanberg, and C. Kuhn. 2004. Prepartum, postpartum, and chronic depression effects on newborns. *Psychiatry* 67 (1):63–80.

Dimidjian, S., S. D. Hollon, K. S. Dobson, K. B. Schmaling, R. J. Kohlenberg, M. E. Addis, et al. 2006. Randomized trial of behavioral activation, cognitive therapy, and antidepressant medication in the acute treatment of adults with major depression. *Journal of Consulting and Clinical Psychology* 74 (4):658–670.

Dinges, D. F., M. T. Orne, W. G. Whitehouse, and E. C. Orne. 1987. Temporal placement of a nap for alertness: Contributions of circadian phase and prior wakefulness. *Sleep* 10 (4):313–329.

DiScalea, T. L., B. H. Hanusa, and K. L. Wisner. 2009. Sexual function in postpartum women treated for depression: Results from a randomized trial of Nortriptyline versus Sertraline. *Journal of Clinical Psychiatry* 70 (3):423–428.

Dix, T. 1991. The affective organization of parenting: Adaptive and maladaptative processes. *Psychological Bulletin* 110 (1):3–25.

Doan, T., A. Gardiner, C. L. Gay, and K. A. Lee. 2007. Breast-feeding increases sleep duration of new parents. *The Journal of Perinatal & Neonatal Nursing* 21 (3):200–206.

Dobson, K. S., S. D. Hollon, S. Dimidjian, K. B. Schmaling, R. J. Kohlenberg, R. J. Gallop, S. L. Rizvi, J. K. Gollan, D. L. Dunner, and N. S. Jacobson. 2008. Randomized trial of behavioral activation, cognitive therapy, and antidepressant medication in the prevention of relapse and recurrence in major depression. *Journal of Consulting and Clinical Psychology* 76 (3):468–477.

Doss, B. D., G. K. Rhoades, S. M. Stanley, and H. J. Markman. 2009. The effect of the transition to parenthood on relationship quality: An 8-year prospective study. *Journal of Personality and Social Psychology* 96 (3):601–619.

Dzaja, A., S. Arber, J. Hislop, M. Kerkhofs, C. Kopp, T. Pollmacher, et al. 2005. Women's sleep in health and disease. *Journal of Psychiatric Research* 39 (1):55–76.

Easterlin, R. A. 2001. Income and happiness: Toward a unified theory. *The Economic Journal* 111 (July):465–484.

Ehrensaft, D. 1997. *Spoiling Childhood: How Well-Meaning Parents Are Giving Children Too Much—But Not What They Need.* New York: Guilford Press.

Eigsti, I. M., V. Zayas, W. Mischel, Y. Shoda, O. Ayduk, M. B. Dadlani, M. C. Davidson, J. Lawrence Aber, B.J. Casey. Predicting cognitive control from preschool to late adolescence and young adulthood. *Psychological Science* 17 (6):478-484.

Erikson, E. H. 1950. *Childhood and Society.* New York: W.W. Norton & Company.

Escriba, V., R. Mas, P. Romito, and M. J. Saurel-Cubizolles. 1999. Psychological distress of new Spanish mothers. *European Journal of Public Health* 9 (4):294–299.

Etkin, A., and T. D. Wager. 2007. Functional neuroimaging of anxiety: A meta-analysis of emotional processing in PTSD, social anxiety disorder, and specific phobia. *American Journal of Psychiatry* 164:1476–1488.

Evans, M. D., S. D. Hollon, R. J. DeRubeis, J. M. Piasecki, W. M. Grove, M. J. Garvey, and V. B. Tuason. 1992. Differential relapse following cognitive therapy and pharmacotherapy for depression. *Archives of General Psychiatry* 49 (10):802–808.

Fava, G., C. Rafanelli, S. Grandi, S. Conti, and P. Belluardo. 1998. Prevention of recurrent depression with cognitive behavioral therapy. *Archives of General Psychiatry* 55:816–820.

Federal Bureau of Investigation. 2004. *Crime in the United States 2004: Uniform Crime Reports.* Washington, DC: Federal Bureau of Investigation.

Feinberg, R. A. 1986. Credit cards as spending facilitating stimuli: A conditioning interpretation. *Journal of Consumer Research* 13:348–356.

Feldman, R. 2006. From biological rhythms to social rhythms: Physiological precursors of mother-infant synchrony. *Developmental Psychology* 42 (1):175–188.

Ferber, R. 2006. *Solve Your Child's Sleep Problems: New, Revised, and Expanded Edition.* New York: Fireside.

Ferguson, C. J. 2010. A meta-analysis of normal and disordered personality across the life span. *Journal of Personality and Social Psychology* 98 (4):659–667.

Fernald, A., and H. Morikawa. 1993. Common themes and cultural variations in Japanese and American mothers' speech to infants. *Child Development* 64:637–656.

Field, T., B. T. Healy, S. Goldstein, and M. Guthertz. 1990. Behavior-state matching and synchrony in mother-infant interactions of nondepressed versus depressed dyads. *Developmental Psychology* 26 (1):7–14.

Figueiredo, B., T. Field, M. Diego, M. Hernandez-Reif, O. Deeds, and A. Ascencio. 2008. Partner relationships during the transition to parenthood. *Journal of Reproductive and Infant Psychology* 26 (2):99–107.

Fisher, D. 1922. Aren't you glad you're not your grandmother? *Good Housekeeping*, April 1922, 28–29.

Fisher, I. 1928. *The Money Illusion*. Binghamton, NY: Vail-Ballou Press Inc.

Fowler, J. H., and N. A. Christakis. 2008. Dynamic spread of happiness in a large social network: Longitudinal analysis over 20 years in the Framingham Heart Study. *British Medical Journal* 337 (2338).

Fox, G. L., C. Bruce, and T. Combs-Orme. 2000. Parenting expectations and concerns of fathers and mothers of newborn infants. *Family Relations* 49 (2):123–131.

Freeman, J. B., N. O. Rule, N. Ambady, and Y. C. Joan. 2009. The cultural neuroscience of person perception. In *Progress in Brain Research*, edited by J. Chiao. Maryland Heights, MO: Elsevier Science.

Frijda, N. H. 1988. The laws of emotion. *American Psychologist* 43 (5):349–358.

Frohlich, P., and C. M. Meston. 2005. Fluoxetine-induced changes in tactile sensation and sexual functioning among clinically depressed women. *Journal of Sex & Marital Therapy* 31 (2):113–128.

Fulcher, M., E. L. Sutfin, R. W. Chan, J. E. Scheib, and C. J. Patterson. 2006. Lesbian mothers and their children: Findings from the contemporary families study. In *Sexual Orientation and Mental Health: Examining Identity and Development in Lesbian, Gay, and Bisexual People*, edited by A. M. Omoto and H. S. Kurtzman. Washington, DC: American Psychological Association.

Gage, G., and D. Christensen. 1991. Parental role socialization and the transition to parenthood. *Family Relations* 40:332–337.

Galinsky, E., K. Aumann, and J. T. Bond. 2009. *Times are Changing: Gender and Generation at Work and at Home*. New York: Families and Work Institute.

Gallant, S. J., J. A. Hamilton, D. A. Popiel, P. J. Morokoff, and P. K. Chakraborty. 1991. Daily moods and symptoms: Effects of awareness of study focus, gender, menstrual-cycle phase, and day of the week. *Health Psychology* 10 (3):180–189.

Gallese, V. 2003. The roots of empathy: the shared manifold hypothesis and the neural basis of intersubjectivity. *Psychopathology* 36 (4):171–180.

Galli, N., and J. J. Reel. 2009. Adonis or Hephaestus? Exploring body image in male athletes. *Psychology of Men & Masculinity* 10 (2):95–108.

Gay, C. L., K. A. Lee, and S.-Y. Lee. 2004. Sleep patterns and fatigue in new mothers and fathers. *Biological Research for Nursing* 5 (4):311–318.

Gianaros, P. J., J. A. Horenstein, S. Cohen, K. A. Matthews, S. M. Brown, J. D. Flory, H. D. Critchley, S. B. Manuck, and A. R. Hariri. 2007. Perigenual anterior cingulate morphology covaries with perceived social standing. *Social Cognitive and Affective Neuroscience* 2:161–173.

Gianino, M. 2008. Adaptation and transformation: The transition to adoptive parenthood for gay male couples. *Journal of GLBT Family Studies* 4 (2):205–243.

Giesler, R. B., R. A. Josephs, and W. B. Swann Jr. 1996. Self-verification in clinical depression: The desire for negative evaluation. *Journal of Abnormal Psychology* 105 (3):358–368.

Gilbert, D. 2005a. Exploring the frontiers of happiness. http://blog.ted.com/2008/12/exploring_the_f.php.

Gilbert, D. 2005b. *Stumbling on Happiness.* New York: Vintage Books.

Gilbert, D. 2009. What you don't know makes you nervous. *New York Times,* May 20, 2009.

Gjerdingen, D. K., and B. A. Center. 2005. The relationship of postpartum partner satisfaction to parents' work, health, and social characteristics. *Women and Health* 40 (4):24–40.

Gladwell, M. 2000. *The Tipping Point: How Little Things Can Make a Big Difference.* New York: Little, Brown, and Company.

Gladwell, M. 2008. *Outliers: The Story of Success.* New York: Little, Brown, and Company.

Goldberg, A. E., and M. Perry-Jenkins. 2004. Division of labor and working-class women's well-being across the transition to parenthood. *Journal of Family Psychology* 18 (1):225–236.

Goldberg, A. E., and A. Sayer. 2006. Lesbian couples' relationship quality across the transition to parenthood. *Journal of Marriage and Family* 68:87–100.

Goode, E. 2000. How culture molds habits of thought. *New York Times*, August 8.

Goodenough, D. R., A. Shapiro, M. Holden, and L. Steinschriber. 1959. A comparison of "dreamers" and "nondreamers": Eye movements, electro-encephalograms, and the recall of dreams. *The Journal of Abnormal and Social Psychology* 59 (3):295–302.

Goodman, J. H. 2004. Paternal postpartum depression, its relationship to maternal postpartum depression, and implications for family health. *Journal of Advanced Nursing* 45 (1):26–35.

Gourville, J. T. 1998. Pennies-a-day: The effect of temporal reframing on transaction evaluation. *Journal of Consumer Research* 24:395–408.

Goyal, D., C. L. Gay, and K. A. Lee. 2007. Patterns of sleep disruption and depressive symptoms in new mothers. *Journal of Perinatal and Neonatal Nursing* 21 (2):123–9.

Goyal, D., C. L. Gay, and K. A. Lee. 2009. Fragmented maternal sleep is more strongly correlated with depressive symptoms than infant temperament at three months postpartum. *Archives of Women's Mental Health* 12 (4):229–237.

Greenberg, G. 2010. *Manufacturing Depression: The Secret History of a Modern Disease*. New York: Simon & Schuster.

Greenstein, T. N. 2000. Economic dependence, gender and the division of labor in the home: A replication and extension. *Journal of Marriage & the Family* 62 (2):322–335.

Gross, J. J. 1998. The emerging field of emotion regulation: An integrative review. *Review of General Psychology* 2 (3):271–299.

Grote, N. K., and M. S. Clark. 2001. Perceiving unfairness in the family: Cause or consequence of marital distress? *Journal of Personality and Social Psychology* 80 (2):281–293.

Gursky, J. T., and L. F. Krahn. 2000. The effects of antidepressants on sleep: A review. *Harvard Review of Psychiatry* 8 (6):298–306.

Hackel, L. S., and D. N. Ruble. 1992. Changes in the marital relationship after the first baby is born: Predicting the impact of expectancy disconfirmation. *Journal of Personality and Social Psychology* 62 (6):944–957.

Haeffel, G. J., B. E. Gibb, G. I. Metalsky, L. B. Alloy, L. Y. Abramson, B. L. Hankin, T. E. Joiner Jr., and J. D. Swedsen. 2008. Measuring cognitive vulnerability to depression: Development and validation of the cognitive style questionnaire. *Clinical Psychology Review* 28:824–836.

Haeffel, G. J., Z. R. Voelz, and T. E. Joiner Jr. 2007. Vulnerability to depressive symptoms: Clarifying the role of excessive reassurance seeking and perceived social support in an interpersonal model of depression. *Cognition & Emotion* 21 (3):681–688.

Hargreaves, D. A., and M. Tiggemann. 2009. Muscular ideal media images and men's body image: Social comparison processing and individual vulnerability. *Psychology of Men & Masculinity* 10 (2):109–119.

Harkness, S. 1987. The cultural mediation of postpartum depression. *Medical Anthropology Quarterly* 1:194–209.

Harrington, B., F. Van Deusen, and J. Ladge. The New Dad: Exploring fatherhood within a career context. Boston College Center for Work and Family, 2010.

Hartley, C. A., and E. A. Phelps. 2009. Changing fear: The neurocircuity of emotion regulation. *Neuropsychopharmacology* **35 (1)**:136–146.

Harwood, K., N. McLean, and K. Durkin. 2007. First-time mothers' expectations of parenthood: What happens when optimistic expectations are not matched by later experiences? *Developmental Psychology* 43 (1):1–12.

Haven, T. J., and L. A. Pearlman. 2004. Minding the body: The intersection of dissociation and physical health in relational trauma psychotherapy. In *Health Consequences of Abuse in the Family: A Clinical Guide for Evidence-Based Practice*, edited by K. A. Kendall-Tackett. Washington, DC: American Psychological Association.

Hefferon, K., M. Grealy, and N. Mutrie. 2009. Post-traumatic growth and life threatening physical illness: A systematic review of the qualitative literature. *British Journal of Health Psychology* 14 (2):343–378.

Hertenstein, M. J., R. Holmes, M. McCullough, and D. Keltner. 2009. The communication of emotion via touch. *Emotion* 9 (4):566–573.

Hirschman, E. C. 1979. Differences in consumer purchase behavior by credit card payment system. *Journal of Consumer Research* 6:58–66.

Hollon, S. D., R. J. DeRubeis, R. C. Shelton, J. D. Amsterdam, R. M. Salomon, J. P. O'Reardon, et al. 2005. Prevention of relapse following cognitive therapy vs. medications in moderate to severe depression. *Archives of General Psychiatry* 62 (4):417–422.

Hoon, P. W., J. P. Wincze, and E. F. Hoon. 1977. A test of reciprocal inhibition: Are anxiety and sexual arousal in women mutually inhibitory? *Journal of Abnormal Psychology* 86 (1):65–74.

Iacoboni, M., and M. Dapretto. 2006. The mirror neuron system and the consequences of its dysfunction. *Nature Reviews: Neuroscience* 7 (12):942–951.

Iacoboni, M., and J. C. Mazziotta. 2007. Mirror neuron system: Basic findings and clinical applications. *Annals of Neurology* 62 (3):213–218.

Ishii-Kuntz, M., and K. Seccombe. 1989. The impact of children upon social support networks throughout the life course. *Journal of Marriage & the Family* 51 (3):777–790.

Joiner, T. E. 1994. Contagious depression: Existence, specificity to depressed symptoms, and the role of reassurance seeking. *Journal of Personality and Social Psychology* 67 (2):287–296.

Joiner, T. E. 1995. The price of soliciting and receiving negative feedback: Self-verification theory as a vulnerability to depression theory. *Journal of Abnormal Psychology* 104 (2):364–372.

Joormann, J., M. Dkane, and I. H. Gotlib. 2006. Adaptive and maladaptive components of rumination? Diagnostic specificity and relation to depressive biases. *Behavior Therapy* 37 (3):269–280.

Kagan, J. 1996. Three pleasing ideas. *American Psychologist* 51 (9):901–908.

Kagan, J. 1997. Family experience and the child's development. In *The Evolution of Psychology: Fifty Years of the American Psychologist*. Edited by J. M. Notterman. Washington, DC: American Psychological Association.

Kagan, J. 2000. Temperament. In *Encyclopedia of Psychology, vol. 8*, edited by A. E. Kazdin. Washington, DC: American Psychological Association.

Kagan, J., D. Arcus, and N. Snidman. 1993. The idea of temperament: Where do we go from here? In *Nature, Nurture, and Psychology*, edited by R. Plomin and G. E. McClearn. Washington, DC: American Psychological Association.

Kagan, J., D. Arcus, N. Snidman, W. Y. Feng, J. Hendler, and S. Greene. 1994. Reactivity in infants: A cross-national comparison. *Developmental Psychology* 30 (3):342–345.

Kagan, J., J. S. Reznick, and N. Snidman. 1988. Biological bases of childhood shyness. *Science* 240 (4849):167–171.

Kahn-Greene, E. T., E. L. Lipizzi, A. K. Conrad, G. H. Kamimori, and W. D. S. Killgore. 2006. Sleep deprivation adversely affects interpersonal responses to frustration. *Personality and Individual Differences* 41 (8):1433–1443.

Katz, J., and T. E. Joiner Jr. 2001. The aversive interpersonal context of depression: Emerging perspectives on depressotypic behavior. In *Behaving Badly: Aversive Behaviors in Interpersonal Relationships*, edited by R. M. Kowalski. Washington, DC: American Psychological Association.

Kennedy, H. P., A. Gardiner, C. L. Gay, and K. A. Lee. 2007. Negotiating sleep: A qualitative study of new mothers. *The Journal of Perinatal & Neonatal Nursing* 21 (2):114–122.

King, L. A., and J. A. Hicks. 2007. Whatever happened to "What might have been"? Regrets, happiness, and maturity. *American Psychologist* 62 (7):625–636.

King-Casas, B., C. Sharp, L. Lomax-Bream, T. Lohrenz, P. Fonagy, and P. R. Montague. 2008. The rupture and repair of cooperation in borderline personality disorder. *Science* 321 (5890):806–810.

Kirsch, I., ed. 1999. *How Expectancies Shape Experience*. Washington, DC: American Psychological Association.

Kirsch, I. 2010. *The Emperor's New Drugs: Exploding the Antidepressant Myth*. New York: Basic Books.

Kit, L. K., G. Janet, and R. Jegasothy. 1997. Incidence of postnatal depression in Malaysian women. *The Journal of Obstetrics and Gynaecology Research* 23:85–89.

Kitayama, S., H. Park, A. T. Sevincer, M. Karasawa, and A. K. Uskul. 2009. A cultural task analysis of implicit independence: Comparing North America, Western Europe, and East Asia. *Journal of Personality and Social Psychology* 97 (2):236–255.

Klein, H. 1991. Couvade syndrome: Male counterpart to pregnancy. *International Journal of Psychiatry in Medicine* 21 (1):57–69.

Kleinman, A., and B. Good, eds. 1985. *Culture and Depression*. Berkeley, CA: University of California Press.

Kluwer, E. S., and M. D. Johnson. 2007. Conflict frequency and relationship quality across the transition to parenthood. *Journal of Marriage and Family* 69 (5):1089–1106.

Knott, J. R., F. A. Gibbs, and C. E. Henry. 1942. Fourier transforms of the electroencephalogram during sleep. *Journal of Experimental Psychology* 31 (6):465–477.

Kozak, M., H. Frankenhauser, and T. A. Roberts. 2009. Objects of desire: Objectification as a function of male sexual orientation. *Psychology of Men & Masculinity* 10 (3):225–230.

Kraus, M. W., and S. Chen. 2009. Striving to be known by significant others: Automatic activation of self-verification goals in relationship contexts. *Journal of Personality and Social Psychology* 97 (1):58–73.

Kross, E., O. Ayduk, and W. Mischel. 2006. When asking "Why" does not hurt: Distinguishing rumination from reflective processing of negative emotions. *Psychological Science* 16 (9):709–717.

Kuffel, S. W., and J. R. Heiman. 2006. Effects of depressive symptoms and experimentally adopted schemas on sexual arousal and affect in sexually healthy women. *Archives of Sexual Behavior* 35 (2):163–177.

Kumar, A. A., J. M. Calheiros, E. Matos, and E. Figueiredo. 1996. Post-natal depression in an urban area of Portugal: Comparison of childbearing women and matched controls. *Psychological Medicine* 26:135–141.

Kumari, V. 2006. Do psychotherapies produce neurobiological effects? *Acta Neuropsychiatrica* 18:61–70.

Landsness, E. C., D. Crupi, B. K. Hulse, M. J. Peterson, R. Huber, H. Ansari, et al. 2009. Sleep-dependent improvement in visuomotor learning: A causal role for slow waves. *Sleep: Journal of Sleep and Sleep Disorders Research* 32 (10):1273–1284.

LaRossa, R. 1983. The transition to parenthood and the social reality of time. *Journal of Marriage & the Family* 45 (3):579–589.

LaRossa, R. 1988. Fatherhood and social change. *Family Relations* 37 (4):451–457.

Lavender, A., and E. Watkins. 2004. Rumination and future thinking in depression. *British Journal of Clinical Psychology* 43 (2):129–142.

Lawrence, B., and H. W. Smith. 1897. *The Practice of the Presence of God: Conversations & Letters of Nicholas Herman of Lorraine.* Translated by H. W. Smith. Seattle, WA: Eremitical Press.

Lawrence, E., R. J. Cobb, A. D. Rothman, M. T. Rothman, and T. N. Bradbury. 2008. Marital satisfaction across the transition to parenthood. *Journal of Family Psychology* 22 (1):41–50.

Lawrence, E., K. Nylen, and R. J. Cobb. 2007. Prenatal expectations and marital satisfaction over the transition to parenthood. *Journal of Family Psychology* 21 (2):155–164.

Lazar, S. W., C. E. Kerr, R. H. Wasserman, J. R. Gray, D. N. Greve, M. T. Treadway, et al. 2005. Meditation experience is associated with increased cortical thickness. *NeuroReport* 16 (17):1893–1897.

Leathers, S. J., M. A. Kelley, and J. A. Richman. 1997. Postpartum depressive symptomatology in new mothers and fathers: Parenting, work, and support. *Journal of Nervous and Mental Disease* 185(3):129–139.

LeBon, O. 2005. Contribution of sleep research to the development of new antidepressants. *Dialogues in Clinical Neuroscience* 7 (4):305–313.

Lee, D. T. S., A. S. K. Yip, H. F. K. Chiu, T. Y. S. Leung, and T. K. H. Chung. 2001. A psychiatric epidemiological study of postpartum Chinese women. *American Journal of Psychiatry* 158:220–226.

Lehrer, J. 2009. Don't. *New Yorker Magazine*, May 18. http://www.newyorker.com/reporting/2009/05/18/090518fa_fact_lehrer.

Leproult R., and E. Van Cauter. 2010. Role of sleep and sleep loss in hormonal release and metabolism. *Endocrine Development* 17:11–21.

Leung, P., S. Erich, and H. Kanenberg. 2005. A comparison of family functioning in gay/lesbian, heterosexual and special needs adoptions. *Children and Youth Services Review* 27 (9):1031–1044.

LeVine, R. A., and R. S. New, eds. 2008. *Anthropology and Child Development: A Cross Cultural Reader*. Malden, MA: Blackwell Publishing.

Levitski, S., and R. Cooper. 2000. Infant colic syndrome: Maternal fantasies of aggression and infanticide. *Clinical Pediatrics* 39:395–400.

Liabsuetrakul, T., A. Vittayanont, and J. Pitanupong. 2007. Clinical applications of anxiety, social support, stressors, and self-esteem measured during pregnancy and postpartum for screening postpartum depression in Thai women. *The Journal of Obstetrics and Gynaecology Research* 33 (3):333–340.

Linehan, M. 1993a. *Cognitive-Behavioral Treatment of Borderline Personality Disorder*. New York: Guilford Press.

Linehan, M. 1993b. *Skills Training Manual for Treating Borderline Personality Disorder*. New York: Guilford Press.

Lipkin, M., and G. S. Lamb. 1982. The couvade syndrome: An epidemiologic study. *Annals of Internal Medicine* 96:509–511.

Liston, C., B. S. McEwen, and B. J. Casey. 2008. Psychosocial stress reversibly disrupts prefrontal processing and attentional control. *Proceedings of the National Academy of Sciences of the United States of America*.

Lobaugh, E. R., P. T. Clements, J. B. Averill, and D. L. Olguin. 2006. Gay-male couples who adopt: Challenging historical and contemporary social trends toward becoming a family. *Perspectives in Psychiatric Care* 42 (3):184–195.

Longsdon, M. C., A. B. McBride, and J. C. Birkhimer. 1994. Social support and postpartum depression. *Research in Nursing and Health* 17:449–457.

LoPiccolo, J., and L. LoPiccolo. 1978. *Handbook of Sex Therapy.* New York.

LoPiccolo, J., and W. E. Stock. 1986. Treatment of sexual dysfunction. *Journal of Consulting and Clinical Psychology* 54 (2):158–167.

Lutz, A., L. G. Lawrence, N. B. Rawlings, M. Ricard, and R. J. Davidson. 2004. Long-term meditators self-induce high-amplitude gamma synchrony during mental practice. *Proceedings of the National Academy of Sciences of the United States of America* 101 (46):16369–16373.

Lyubomirsky, S., and S. Nolen-Hoeksema. 1995. Effects of self-focused rumination on negative thinking and interpersonal problem solving. *Journal of Personality and Social Psychology* 69 (1):176–190.

Lyubomirsky, S., K. L. Tucker, N. D. Caldwell, and K. Berg. 1999. Why ruminators are poor problem solvers: Clues from the phenomenology of dysphoric rumination. *Journal of Personality and Social Psychology* 77 (5):1041–1060.

Madanes, C., and C. Madanes. 1994. *The Secret Meaning of Money: How to Prevent Financial Problems from Destroying Our Most Intimate Relationships.* San Francisco, CA: Jossey-Bass.

Marsella, A. J., N. Sartorius, A. Jablensy, and F. R. Fenton. 1985. Cross-cultural studies of depressive disorders: An overview. In *Culture and Depression: Studies in the Anthropology and Cross-Cultural Psychiatry of Affect and Disorder,* edited by A. Kleinman and B. Good. Berkeley, CA: University of California Press.

MacDermid, S., T. Huston, and S. McHale. 1990. Changes in marriage associated with the transition to parenthood: Individual differences as a function of sex-role attitudes and changes in the division of household labor. *Journal of Marriage & the Family* 52:475–486.

Markman, H. J., S. M. Stanley, and S. L. Blumberg. 2001. *Fighting for Your Marriage: Positive Steps for Preventing Divorce and Preserving a Lasting Love (New & Revised).* New York: John Wiley & Sons.

Marks, S. 1979. Culture, human energy, and self-actualization: A sociological offering to humanistic psychology. *Journal of Humanistic Psychology* 19 (3):27-42.

Marks, S. R. 1977. Multiple roles and role strain: Some notes on human energy, time, and commitment. *American Sociological Review* 42 (6):921–936.

Marshall, G. N., T. L. Schell, and J. N. V. Miles. 2009. Ethnic differences in posttraumatic distress: Hispanics' symptoms differ in kind and degree. *Journal of Consulting and Clinical Psychology* 77 (6):1169–1178.

Maslow, A. H. 1962. *Toward a Psychology of Being.* New York: Wiley and Sons.

Mason, C., and R. Elwood. 1995. Is there a physiological basis for the couvade and onset of paternal care? *International Journal of Nursing Studies* 32 (2):137–148.

Masuda, T., and R. E. Nisbett. 2001. Attending holistically versus analytically: Comparing the context sensitivity of Japanese and Americans. *Journal of Personality and Social Psychology* 81 (5):922–934.

McCarthy, B., and E. McCarthy. 2003. *Rekindling Desire: A Step-by-Step Program to Help Low-Sex and No-Sex Marriages.* New York: Brunner-Routledge.

McCarthy, B., and M. Thestrup. 2009. Men, intimacy, and eroticism. *Journal of Sexual Medicine* 6:588–594.

McEwen, B. S. 2009. The brain is the central organ of stress and adaptation. *Neuroimage* 47:911–913.

McHale, J. P., C. Kazali, T. Rotman, J. Talbot, M. Carleton, and R. Lieberson. 2004. The transition to coparenthood: Parents' prebirth expectations and early coparental adjustment at 3 months postpartum. *Development and Psychopathology* 16:711–733.

McKay, M., P. Fanning, and K. Paleg. 2006. *Couple Skills: Making Your Relationship Work.* Oakland, CA: New Harbinger Publications.

McNulty, J. K., and B. R. Karney. 2004. Positive expectations in the early years of marriage: Should couples expect the best or brace for the worst? *Journal of Personality and Social Psychology* 86 (5):729–743.

Medina, A. M., C. L. Lederhos, and T. A. Lillis. 2009. Sleep disruption and decline in marital satisfaction across the transition to parenthood. *Families, Systems, & Health* 27 (2):153–160.

Meignan, M., M. W. Davis, S. P. Thomas, and P. G. Droppleman. 1999. Living with postpartum depression: The father's experience. *The American Journal of Maternal Child Nursing* 24:202–208.

Meiser-Stedman, R., T. Dalgleish, E. Glucksman, W. Yule, and P. Smith. 2009. Maladaptive cognitive appraisals mediate the evolution of posttraumatic stress reactions: A 6-month follow-up of child and adolescent assault and motor vehicle accident survivors. *Journal of Abnormal Psychology* 118 (4):778–787.

Merikangas, K. R., A. Chakravarti, S. O. Moldin, H. Araj, J. Blangero, M. Burmeister, et al. 2002. Workgroup reports: NIMH strategic plan for mood disorders research; future of genetics of mood disorders research. *Biological Psychiatry* 52:457–477.

Meston, C. M., and D. M. Buss. 2007. Why humans have sex. *Archives of Sexual Behavior* 36:477–507.

Middleton, L. S., S. W. Kuffel, and J. R. Heiman. 2008. Effects of experimentally adopted sexual schemas on vaginal response and subjective sexual arousal: A comparison between women with sexual arousal disorder and sexually healthy women. *Archives of Sexual Behavior* 37(6):950–61.

Mischel, W., and C. Gilligan. 1964. Delay of gratification, motivation for the prohibited gratification, and responses to temptation. *The Journal of Abnormal and Social Psychology* 69 (4):411–417.

Monk, T. H., D. J. Buysse, J. Carrier, B. D. Billy, and L. R. Rose. 2001. Effects of afternoon "siesta" naps on sleep, alertness, performance, and circadian rhythms in the elderly. *Sleep* 24 (6):680–687.

Morof, D., G. Barrett, J. Peacock, C. R. Victor, and I. Manyonda. 2003. Postnatal depression and sexual health after childbirth. *Obstetrics and Gynecology* 102 (6):1318–25.

Morse, J. M. 1997. Compathy: The contagion of physical distress. *Journal of Advanced Nursing* 26:649–657.

Murphy, G. 1949. The relationships of culture and personality. In *Culture and personality.* New York: Viking Fund.

Murray, A. 2003. *Abiding in Christ.* Bloomington, MN: Bethany House Publishers.

Muzet, A. 2005. Alteration of sleep microstructure in psychiatric disorders. *Dialogues in Clinical Neuroscience* 7 (Special Issue on sleep):315–321.

Nager, A., L. M. Johansson, and K. Sundquist. 2006. Neighborhood socioeconomic environment and risk of postpartum psychosis. *Archives of Women's Mental Health* 9 (81–86).

Nelson, J., and A. G. Harvey. 2003. An exploration of pre-sleep cognitive activity in insomnia: Imagery and verbal thought. *British Journal of Clinical Psychology* 42 (3):271–288.

Nisbett, R. E., and T. Masuda. 2007. Culture and point of view. *Intellectica* 46–47 (2–3):153–172.

Noh, Y.-H. 2009. Does unemployment increase suicide rates? The OECD panel evidence. *Journal of Economic Psychology* 30:575–582.

Nolen-Hoeksema, S. 1987. Sex differences in unipolar depression: Evidence and theory. *Psychological Bulletin* 101 (2):259–282.

Norenzayan, A., I. Choi, and K. Peng. 2007. Perception and cognition. In *Handbook of Cultural Psychology*, edited by S. Kitayama and D. Cohen. New York: Guilford Press.

O'Hara, M. W., L. P. Rehm, and S. B. Campbell. 1982. Predicting depressive symptomatology: Cognitive-behavioral models and postpartum depression. *Journal of Abnormal Psychology* 91 (6):457–61.

O'Hara, M. W., L. P. Rehm, and S. B. Campbell. 1983. Postpartum depression. A role for social network and life stress variables. *The Journal of Nervous and Mental Disease* 171 (6):336–41.

Okun, M. L., B. H. Hanusa, M. Hall, and K. L. Wisner. 2009. Sleep complaints in late pregnancy and the recurrence of postpartum depression. *Behavioral Sleep Medicine* 7:106–117.

Ophir, E., C. Nass, and A. D. Wagner. 2009. Cognitive control in media multitaskers. In *Proceedings of the National Academy of Sciences of the United States of America.* Washington, DC: National Academy of Sciences.

Pace-Schott, E. F., M. R. Milad, S. P. Orr, S. L. Rauch, R. Stickgold, and R. K. Pitman. 2009. Sleep promotes generalization of extinction of conditioned fear. *Sleep: Journal of Sleep and Sleep Disorders Research* 32 (1):19–26.

Palace, E. M., and B. B. Gorzalka. 1990. The enhancing effects of anxiety on arousal in sexually dysfunctional and functional women. *Journal of Abnormal Psychology* 99 (4):403–411.

Papa, A., and G. A. Bonanno. 2008. Smiling in the face of adversity: The interpersonal and intrapersonal functions of smiling. *Emotion* 8 (1):1–12.

Paquette, V., J. Le´Vesque, B. Mensour, J.-M. Leroux, G. Beaudoin, P. Bourgouin, and M. Beauregard. 2003. ⊠Change the mind and you change the brain⊠: Effects of cognitive behavioral therapy on the neural correlates of spider phobia. *Neuroimage* 18 (2):401–409.

Pastore, L., A. Owens, and C. Raymond. 2007. Postpartum sexuality concerns among first-time parents from one U.S. academic hospital. *Journal of Sexual Medicine* 4:115–123.

Patterson, C. 2000. Family relationships of lesbians and gay men. *Journal of Marriage & the Family* 62 (4):1052–1070.

Pauls, R. N., J. A. Occhino, and V. L. Dryfhout. 2008. Effects of pregnancy on female sexual function and body image: A prospective study. *Journal of Sexual Medicine* 5 (8):1915–1922.

Pauls, R. N., J. A. Occhino, V. L. Dryfhout, and M. Karram. 2008. Effects of pregnancy on pelvic floor dysfunction and body image; a prospective study. *International Urogynecology Journal* 19:1495–1501.

Paulson, J. F., S. Dauber, and J. A. Leiferman. 2006. Individual and combined effects of postpartum depression in mothers and fathers on parenting behavior. *Pediatrics* 118 (2):659–668.

Paulson, J. F., H. A. Keefe, and J. A. Leiferman. 2009. Early parental depression and child language development. *Journal of Child Psychology and Psychiatry* 50 (3):254–262.

Peng, K., and R. E. Nisbett. 1999. Culture, dialectics, and reasoning about contradiction. *American Psychologist* 54 (9):741–754.

Perel, E. 2007. *Mating in Captivity: Unlocking Erotic Intelligence.* New York: Harper.

Peterson, M., and J. F. Wilson. 2004. Work stress in America. *International Journal of Stress Management* 11 (2):91–113.

Pettit, J. W., and T. E. Joiner. 2006a. Excessive reassurance-seeking. In *Chronic Depression: Interpersonal Sources, Therapeutic Solutions.* Washington, DC: American Psychological Association.

Pettit, J. W., and T. E. Joiner. 2006b. Negative feedback-seeking. In *Chronic Depression: Interpersonal Sources, Therapeutic Solutions.* Washington, DC: American Psychological Association.

Pillsbury, B. L. K. 1978. Doing the month: Confinement and convalescence of Chinese women after childbirth. *Social Science and Medicine* 12:11–22.

Potthoff, J. G., C. J. Holahan, and T. E. Joiner. 1995. Reassurance seeking, stress generation, and depressive symptoms: An integrative model. *Journal of Personality and Social Psychology* 68 (4):664–670.

Prelec, D., and G. Loewenstein. 1998. The red and the black: Mental accounting of savings and debt. *Marketing Science* 17: 4–28.

Prelec, D., and D. Simester. 2001. Always leave home without it: A further investigation of the credit-card effect on willingness to pay. *Marketing Letters* 12:5–12.

Purdy, D., and E. Frank. 1993. Should postpartum mood disorders be given a more prominent or distinct place in the DSM-IV? *Depression* 1 (1):59–70.

Radley, J. J., H. M. Sisti, J. Hao, A. B. Rocher, T. McCall, P. R. Hof, B. S. McEwen, and J. H. Morrison. 2004. Chronic behavioral stress induces apical dendritic reorganization in pyramidal neurons of the medial prefrontal cortex. *Neuroscience* 125:1–6.

Rallis, S., H. Skouteris, E. H. Wertheim, and S. J. Paxton. 2007. Predictors of body image during the first year postpartum: A prospective study. *Women & Health* 45 (1):87–104.

Ranson, G. 2001. Men at work: Change—or no change? —in the era of the "New Father." *Men and Masculinities* 4 (1):3–26.

Ravitz, P. 2003. The interpersonal fulcrum: Interpersonal therapy for treatment of depression. *CPA Bulletin* 36 (1):15–19.

Riemann, D., C. Kloepfer, and M. Berger. 2009. Functional and structural brain alterations in insomnia: implications for pathophysiology. *European Journal of Neuroscience* 29:1754–1760.

Risch, N., R. Herrell, T. Lehner, K. Y. Liang, L. Eaves, J. Hoh, A. Griem, M. Kovacs, J. Ott, and K. R. Merikangas. 2009. Interaction between the serotonin transporter gene (5-HTTLPR), stressful life events, and risk of depression: A meta-analysis. *Journal of the American Medical Association* 301 (June 17):2462–2471.

Rizzolatti, G., and L. Craighero. 2004. The mirror neuron system. *Annual Review of Neuroscience* 27:169–192.

Roche, T. 2002. Andrea Yates: More to the story. *Time Magazine*, March 18, 2002.

Romito, P., M. J. Sauren-Cubizolles, and N. Lelong. 1999. What makes new mothers unhappy: psychological distress one year after birth in Italy and France. *Social Science and Medicine* 49:1651–1661.

Sanchez, L., and E. Thomson. 1997. Becoming mothers and fathers: parenthood, gender, and the division of labor. *Gender and Society* 11 (6):747–772.

Sanford, K. 2006. Communication during marital conflict: When couples alter their appraisal, they change their behavior. *Journal of Family Psychology* 20 (2):256–265.

Schulz, M. S., C. P. Cowan, and P. A. Cowan. 2006. Promoting healthy beginnings: A randomized controlled trial of a preventive intervention to preserve marital quality during the transition to parenthood. *Journal of Consulting and Clinical Psychology* 74 (1):20–31.

Seal, B. N., and C. M. Meston. 2007. The impact of body awareness on sexual arousal in women with sexual dysfunction. *Journal of Sexual Medicine* 4:990–1000.

Segre, L. S., M. W. O'Hara, S. Arndt, and S. Stuart. 2007. The prevalence of postpartum depression: The relative significance of three social status indices. *Social Psychiatry and Psychiatric Epidemiology* 42 (4):316–21.

Seligman, M. 1990. *Learned Optimism.* New York: Alfred A. Knopf.

Senecky, Y., H. Agassi, D. Inbar, N. Horesh, G. Diamond, Y. S. Bergman, and A. Apter. 2009. Post-adoption depression among adoptive mothers. *Journal of Affective Disorders* 115 (1–2):62–68.

Shafir, E., P. Diamond, and A. Tversky. 1997. Money illusion. *Quarterly Journal of Economics* 112:341–374.

Shansky, R. M., C. Hamo, P. R. Hof, B. S. McEwen, and J. H. Morrison. 2009. Stress-induced dendritic remodeling in the prefrontal cortex is circuit specific. *Cerebral Cortex* 19(10):2479–84.

Shapiro, A. F., J. M. Gottman, and S. Carrère. 2000. The baby and the marriage: Identifying factors that buffer against decline in marital satisfaction after the first baby arrives. *Journal of Family Psychology* 14 (1):59–70.

Shapiro, S., and J. Nass. 1986. Postpartum psychosis in the male. *Psychopathology* 19 (3):138–142.

Sharma, V., A. Smith, and M. Khan. 2004. The relationship between duration of labour, time of delivery, and puerperal psychosis. *Journal of Affective Disorders* 83 (2–3):215–220.

Shrewsbury, V. A., K. A. Robb, C. Power, and J. Wardle. 2009. Socioeconomic differences in weight retention, weight-related attitudes and practices in postpartum women. *Maternal & Child Health Journal* 13 (2):231–240.

Siegel, J. M. 2009. Sleep viewed as a state of adaptive inactivity. *Nature Reviews Neuroscience* 10 (10):747–753.

Signorello, L. B., B. L. Harlow, A. K. Chekos, and J. T. Repke. 2001. Postpartum sexual functioning and its relationship to perineal trauma: A retrospective cohort study of primiparous women. *American Journal of Obstetrics and Gynecology* 184 (5):881–888.

Simon, G. E., M. Fleck, R. Lucas, and D. M. Bushnell. 2004. Prevalence and predictors of depression treatment in an international primary care study. *American Journal of Psychiatry* 161 (9):1626–1634.

Simon, G. E., D. P. Goldberg, M. Von Korff, and T. B. Üstün. 2002. Understanding cross-national differences in depression prevalence. *Psychological Medicine* 32 (4):585–594.

Singley, S. G., and K. Hynes. 2005. Transitions to parenthood: Work-family policies, gender, and the couple context. *Gender and Society* 19:376–397.

Sohr-Preston, S. L., and L. V. Scaramella. 2006. Implications of timing of maternal depressive symptoms for early cognitive and language development. *Clinical Child and Family Psychology Review* 9 (1):65–83.

Soman, D. 2003. The effect of payment transparency on consumption: Quasi-experiments from the field. *Marketing Letters* 14:173–183.

Spiegel, K., E. Tasali, R. Leproult, and E. Van Cauter. 2009. Effects of poor and short sleep on glucose metabolism and obesity risk. *Nature Reviews: Endocrinology* 5 (5):253–261.

Srivastava, J., and P. Raghubir. 2002. Debiasing using decomposition: The case of memory-based credit card expense estimates. *Journal of Consumer Psychology* 12:253–264.

Stanley, S. M., G. K. Rhoades, and H. J. Markman. 2006. Sliding versus deciding: Inertia and the premarital cohabitation effect. *Family Relations* 55:499–509.

Stanley, S. M., S. W. Whitton, and H. J. Markman. 2004. Maybe I do: Interpersonal commitment and premarital or nonmarital cohabitation. *Journal of Family Issues* 25:496–519.

Starr, L. R., and J. Davila. 2008. Excessive reassurance seeking, depression, and interpersonal rejection: A meta-analytic review. *Journal of Abnormal Psychology* 117 (4):762–775.

Stemp, P. S., R. J. Turner, and S. Noh. 1986. Psychological distress in the post-partum period: The significance of social support. *Journal of Marriage and Family* 48 (2):271–277.

Stern, G., and L. Kruckman. 1983. Multi-disciplinary perspectives on post-partum depression: An anthropological critique. *Social Science and Medicine* (17):1027–1041.

Stix, G. 1996. Listening to culture. *Scientific American* 274 (1).

Storey, A. E., C. J. Walsh, R. L. Quinton, and K. E. Wynne-Edwards. 2000. Hormonal correlates of paternal responsiveness in new and expectant fathers. *Evolution and Human Behavior* 21:79–95.

Sullivan, H. S. 1955. *The Interpersonal Theory of Psychiatry*. London: Tavistock Publications Limited.

Swain, A. M., M. W. O'Hara, K. R. Starr, and L. L. Gorman. 1997. A prospective study of sleep, mood, and cognitive function in postpartum and non-postpartum women. *Obstetrics and Gynecology* 90 (3):381–6.

Swann Jr., W. B., and J. K. Bosson. 1999. The flip side of the reassurance-seeking coin: The partner's perspective. *Psychological Inquiry* 10 (4):302–304.

Tach, L., and S. Halpern-Meekin. 2009. How does premarital cohabitation affect trajectories of marital quality? *Journal of Marriage and Family* 71 (May):298–317.

Takahashi M., H. Fukuda, and H. Arito. 1998. Brief naps during post-lunch rest: Effects on alertness, performance, and autonomic balance. *European Journal of Applied Physiology and Occupational Physiology* 78 (2):93–98.

Tangney, J.P., P.E. Wagner, D. Hill-Barlow, D. E. Marschall, R. Gramzow. 1996. Relation of shame and guilt to constructive versus destructive responses to anger across the lifespan. *Journal of Personality and Social Psychology* 70 (4):797-809.

Tavris, C., and E. Aaronson. 2007. *Mistakes Were Made (but Not by Me): Why We Justify Foolish Beliefs, Bad Decisions, and Hurtful Acts.* New York: Harcourt Inc.

Teasdale, J. D., Z. V. Segal, J. M. G. Williams, V. A. Ridgeway, J. M. Soulsby, and M. A. Lau. 2000. Prevention of relapse/recurrence in major depression by mindfulness-based cognitive therapy. *Journal of Consulting and Clinical Psychology* 68 (4):615–623.

Thase, M. 2006. Depression and sleep: Pathophysiology and treatment. *Dialogues in Clinical Neuroscience* 8 (2):217–226.

Tokunaga, H. 1993. The use and abuse of consumer credit: Applications of psychological theory and research. *Journal of Economic Psychology* 14:285–316.

Trethowan, W. H., and W. F. Conlon. 1965. The couvade syndrome. *British Journal of Psychiatry* 111:57–66.

Twenge, J. 2006. *Generation Me.* New York: Free Press.

Twenge, J. M. 2001. Birth cohort changes in extraversion: A cross-temporal meta-analysis. *Personality and Individual Differences* 30 (5):735–748.

Twenge, J. M., R. F. Baumeister, C. N. DeWall, N. J. Ciarocco, and J. M. Bartels. 2007. Social exclusion decreases prosocial behavior. *Journal of Personality and Social Psychology* 92 (1):56–66.

Twenge, J. M., R. F. Baumeister, D. M. Tice, and T. S. Stucke. 2001. If you can't join them, beat them: Effects of social exclusion on aggressive behavior. *Journal of Personality and Social Psychology* 81 (6):1058–1069.

Twenge, J. M., and W. K. Campbell. 2009. *The Narcissism Epidemic.* New York: Free Press.

Twenge, J. M., W. K. Campbell, and C. A. Foster. 2003. Parenthood and marital satisfaction: A meta-analytic review. *Journal of Marriage and Family* 65 (3):574–583.

Twenge, J. M., K. R. Catanese, and R. F. Baumeister. 2003. Social exclusion and the deconstructed state: Time perception, meaninglessness, lethargy, lack of emotion, and self-awareness. *Journal of Personality and Social Psychology* 85 (3):409–423.

Twenge, J. M., S. Konrath, J. D. Foster, W. K. Campbell, and B. J. Bushman. 2008. Egos inflating over time: A cross-temporal meta-analysis of the narcissistic personality. *Journal of Personality* 76 (4):875–902

Ury, W. 1991. *Getting Past No: Negotiating Your Way from Confrontation to Cooperation.* New York: Bantam Books.

Van Moffaert, M. M. 1994. Sleep disorders and depression: The "chicken and egg" situation. *Journal of Psychosomatic Research* 38 (Supplement 1):9–13.

Van Putten, R., and J. LaWall. 1981. Postpartum psychosis in an adoptive mother and in a father. *Psychosomatics* 22 (12):1087–1089.

von Sydow, K. 1999. Sexuality during pregnancy and after childbirth: A metacontent analysis of 59 studies. *Journal of Psychosomatic Research* 47 (1):27–49.

von Sydow, K. 2002. Sexual enjoyment and orgasm postpartum: Sex differences and perceptual accuracy concerning partners' sexual experience. *Journal of Psychosomatic Obstetrics and Gynaecology* 23 (3):147–155.

Walker, M. P. 2009. The role of sleep in cognition and emotion. *The Year in Cognitive Neuroscience 2009: Annals of the New York Academy of Science* 1156 (Mar):168–197.

Walker, M. P., and E. van der Helm. 2009. Overnight therapy? The role of sleep in emotional brain processing. *Psychological Bulletin* 135 (5):731–748.

Wall, G., and S. Arnold. 2007. How involved is involved fathering?: An exploration of the contemporary culture of fatherhood. *Gender & Society* 21 (4):508–527.

Wang, S. Y., and C. H. Chen. 2006. Psychosocial health of Taiwanese postnatal husbands and wives. *Journal of Psychosomatic Research* 60:303–307.

Watters, E. 2010. *Crazy Like Us: The Globalization of the American Psyche.* New York: Free Press.

Weary, G., J. S. Jordan, and M. G. Hill. 1985. The attributional norm of internality and depressive sensitivity to social information. *Journal of Personality and Social Psychology* 49 (5):1283–1293.

Weber, B., A. Rangel, M. Wibral, and A. Falk. 2009. The medial prefrontal cortex exhibits money illusion. *Proceedings of the National Academy of Sciences of the United States of America* 106 (13):5025–5028.

Wei, G., L. B. Greaver, S. M. Marson, C. H. Herndon, and J. Rogers. 2008. Postpartum depression: Racial differences and ethnic disparities in a tri-racial and bi-ethnic population. *Maternal and Child Health Journal* 12:699–707.

Weisz, J. R., S. Suwanlert, W. Chaiyasit, B. Weiss, B. R. Walter, and W. Wibulswasdi Anderson. 1988. Thai and American perspectives on over- and undercontrolled child behavior problems: Exploring the threshold model among parents, teachers, and psychologists. *Journal of Consulting and Clinical Psychology* 56 (4):601–609.

Wetherell, M. A., M. E. Hyland, and J. E. Harris. 2004. Secretory immuno-globulin A reactivity to acute and cumulative acute multi-tasking stress: Relationships between reactivity and perceived workload. *Biological Psychology* 66 (3):257–270.

Wicks, R. J. 2010. *Bounce: Living the Resilient Life.* New York: Oxford University Press.

Williams, J. M. G., J. D. Teasdale, Z. V. Segal, and J. Soulsby. 2000. Mindfulness-based cognitive therapy reduces overgeneral autobiographical memory in formerly depressed patients. *Journal of Abnormal Psychology* 109 (1):150–155.

World Health Organization. 1999. *The World Health Report 1999: Making a Difference.* Geneva, Switzerland: World Health Organization.

Yapko, M. 1997. *Breaking the Patterns of Depression.* New York: Broadway Books.

Yapko, M. 1999. *Hand Me Down Blues: How to Stop Depression from Spreading in Families.* New York: St. Martins Griffin.

Yapko, M. 2001a. Hypnosis in treating symptoms and risk factors of major depression. *American Journal of Clinical Hypnosis* 44 (2):97–108.

Yapko, M. 2001b. *Treating Depression with Hypnosis: Integrating Cognitive-Behavioral and Strategic Approaches.* Philadelphia: Brunner-Routledge.

Yapko, M. 2009. *Depression Is Contagious.* New York: Free Press.

Zelkowitz, P., and T. H. Milet. 2001. The course of postpartum psychiatric disorders in women and their partners. *Journal of Nervous and Mental Disease* 189:575–582.

Sara Rosenquist, Ph.D., maintains a clinical practice in Chapel Hill, NC, and specializes in reproductive health issues ranging from postpartum depression to sexual dysfunction.

Foreword writer Michael D. Yapko, Ph.D., is a clinical psychologist and marriage and family therapist in Fallbrook, CA. He is author of numerous books, including *Breaking the Patterns of Depression*.

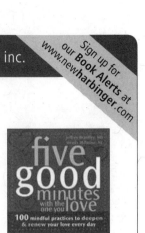
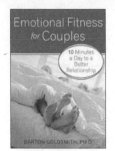
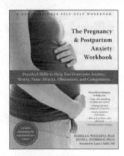
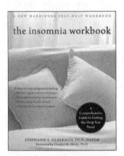
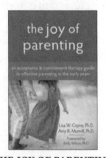
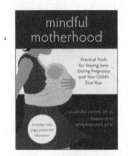